Communication Augmentation

Communication Augmentation: A Casebook of Clinical Management

David R. Beukelman, Ph.D

Kathryn M. Yorkston, Ph.D.

Patricia A. Dowden, M.S.

Communication Augmentation Center
University Affiliated Hospitals
Department of Rehabilitation Medicine
University of Washington, Seattle, Washington

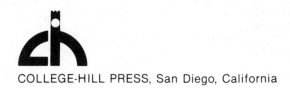

COLLEGE-HILL PRESS, San Diego, California

College-Hill Press, Inc.
4284 41st Street
San Diego, California 92105

Library of Congress Cataloging in Publication Data

Beukelman, David R., 1943–
  Communication augmentation.

  Includes bibliographies and index.
  1. Communicative disorders–Treatment–Case studies. I. Yorkston, Kathryn M.,
1948–   . II. Dowden, Patricia A., 1952–   . III. Title. [DNLM: 1. Nonverbal
Communication–methods–case studies. 2. Speech Disorders–rehabilitation–case
studies. WL 340 B566c]
  RC423.B48   1984   616.85'5   84-15525
  ISBN 0-88744-102-5

Printed in the United States of America

Dedication

Dedicated to our clients
and their families who have been
our primary teachers

TABLE OF CONTENTS

PREFACE

Professionals from many disciplines, including education, physical therapy, occupational therapy, engineering, psychology, and speech-language pathology, are preparing themselves to serve nonspeaking individuals. The need for printed materials to support the continuing education efforts of professionals and the training of students is an important need in the communication augmentation field. However, we found that the task of writing a general textbook was extremely difficult. The field of communication augmentation is extremely complex, with professionals from numerous disciplines providing services to multiple populations across age groups and with disorders of various causations. However, the knowledge base of the field is derived largely from clinical experiences, only a few of which are described in journals containing collections of articles. The education of professionals and students is hampered by the limited availability of clinical observation opportunities because there are few centers that serve a broad range of individuals with severe communicative impairments. Although the research base of the field is growing, it consists primarily of technical reports and a few descriptive reports based on single or multiple case studies.

In *Communication Augmentation: A Casebook Of Clinical Management*, we present the communication augmentation field at several levels. By structuring our discussion around 12 case studies, we introduce the beginning student to nonspeaking individuals of different ages and with disorders of various etiologies. The impact of severe communication disability is described, and interventions are outlined. Through extensive question-and-answer sections at the end of each case study, we review research, technical, clinical, and administrative issues facing the communication augmentation field. The more advanced reader will find intervention programs that reflect up-to-date technology, and training programs that assist our clients to use their communication approaches to meet interpersonal, educational, and vocational needs.

Readers should be aware that this *Casebook* represents the work and therefore the philosophy of a single research and clinical center. However, we have attempted to select cases that represent a range of ages, etiologic conditions, and communicative solutions. We have selected cases whose management has come to some kind of conclusion, although we anticipate we will continue to follow a number of these patients, updating approaches to communication when new technology becomes available or when the user's communication methods need change. In keeping with our effort to present cases which have reached a level of completion, we have chosen to reduce the number of cases highlighting young children, who are in transition. Rather, we are viewing those users with congenital conditions as "children who have grown up." Specific references about serving young children are presented in the *Additional Readings* listed at the conclusion of several chapters. All of the case studies represent the actual experience of the individual described, with one exception, in which the case study is actually a composite of two individuals who presented similar communication needs and intervention strategies. We have not included those cases in which lack of motivation or cooperation has precluded effective intervention.

Chapter 1 provides an overview of the multidisciplinary Communication Augmentation Center located in the Department of Rehabilitation Medicine at the University of Washington, Seattle. In addition, terminology and procedures used throughout the *Casebook* are introduced. Chapters 2 through 13 describe individual case experiences. Six cases involve adults with disorders of sudden onset, including brain-stem hemorrhage, spinal cord injury, laryngectomy-glossectomy, traumatic head injury, and left cerebrovascular accident. Two cases involve adults with amyotrophic lateral sclerosis, a gradual degenerative disease. Finally, four cases involve individuals with cerebral palsy, a disorder present from birth. All case presentation chapters contain background information including age, etiology, social history, and the communication approach used at the beginning of our intervention. Results of our initial evaluation are presented. The phases of intervention, including goal(s), approach(es), and outcome(s), are presented for each case. When appropriate, our case presentations are followed by comments from the users regarding their alternative communication systems. A section entitled *Questions for the Clinician* is included at the conclusion of each case presentation. These discussions allow the clinician to address important issues and serve as a springboard for further discussion. A list of *References* and *Additional Readings* are included at the end of each chapter. Finally, a *Glossary* is provided.

This *Casebook* would not have been completed without considerable support. We acknowledge the help of specific individuals at the end of each chapter. We are especially grateful to Laura McDaniel, who has answered thousands of telephone calls and processed hundreds of funding requests during the past seven years. Bruce Terami has assisted us through the years in providing a photographic record of our center's activities. Carole Lossing is an occupational therapist who served our center for many years. Her contributions are reflected throughout the *Casebook*.

The Pacific Northwest Nonvocal Communication Group, an advocacy group in our area, has supported our center and its staff in many ways. The workshops and seminars sponsored by this group have been a primary educational vehicle for our center's staff. We also wish to thank the network of pioneers in this field who returned most of our calls and sent us most of the pre-prints we requested. Thanks must also go to the staff of the Alternative Communication System Project headed by Wes Wilson. Through them, we learned about the application of Morse code technology to serve the communication needs of the severely physically disabled population. The experiences upon which this *Casebook* is based come from the Communication Augmentation Center located in the Department of Rehabilitation Medicine, University of Washington Hospital, Seattle. The ongoing support from our parent department and hospital has been fundamental to the continuation of our center.

David R. Beukelman, Ph.D
Kathryn M. Yorkston, Ph.D.
Patricia A. Dowden, M.S.

CHAPTER 1

Overview

THE CENTER AND ITS STAFF

In 1977, the Speech-Language Pathology staff of the University of Washington Hospital faced a growing problem: how do we serve the communication needs of nonspeaking individuals? The number of nonspeaking individuals in our caseload was increasing. We were receiving referrals from a variety of sources. The hospital and the Department of Rehabilitation Medicine were beginning to serve increasing numbers of patients with head injuries, some of whom were unable to speak. A staffing change in the Department of Otolaryngology and Head and Neck Surgery resulted in the referral of an increasing number of persons with extensive head and neck cancer to our hospital for their medical care and subsequent rehabilitation programs. For example, patients with simultaneous total glossectomy and total laryngectomy were becoming increasingly common in our caseload. The Departments of Rehabilitation Medicine and Neurology began specialty clinics to serve individuals with amyotrophic lateral sclerosis, Parkinson's disease, and multiple sclerosis, degenerative diseases that often result in severe dysarthria. In short, we were faced with a growing number of individuals in our caseload who could not speak understandably. We realized that supplementation or replacement of speech with communication-alphabet boards and standard electric typewriters was inadequate to meet the needs of these individuals with severe communicative impairments.

Under the sponsorship of the Speech Pathology Unit and the Department of Rehabilitation Medicine, the Augmentative Communication Center was initiated. The core participants included a managing speech-language pathologist, an occupational therapist, an engineering technician, and a secretary. Consulting participants included a physical therapist, rehabilitation physician, neuro-ophthalmologist, psychologist, and computer programmer. The Communication Augmentation Center developed as a functional, rather than administrative, unit with professionals retaining affiliation with their own clinical unit while serving the center as needed. An informal research group was formed to complement the clinical effort. Led by the managing speech-language pathologist, the group included an occupational therapist, several speech-language pathologists, a computer programmer, and a physician. The clinical and research efforts in the communication augmentation area were managed cooperatively. For example, communication equipment needed by the center was purchased using both research and clinical funds. The hospital budgets of the speech pathology, occupational therapy, and engineering application units as well as budgets of research projects provided funds for the purchase of equipment, switches, and mounting systems.   Initially, the center was housed in the speech pathology unit; however, as the program grew, separate space was allocated to the center in conjunction with Computers in Rehabilitation and Brain Injury, a program of the Department of Rehabilitation Medicine.

Through the years from 1977 to early 1984, the role of our center in the educational and medical communities of the Pacific Northwest gradually evolved, until our referrals included patients with a broad range of diagnoses, ages, and capability levels. At this time, the center staff serve as consultants to the medical and educational agencies in the area. In some cases, the consulting agencies provide both thorough evaluations and appropriate intervention and follow-up, while our center serves only as a consultant for technical applications. Other referring agencies have limited resources for dealing with the communication needs of their clients, and our center takes nearly complete responsibility for the client's entire communication program. On occasion, such clients may be admitted to the inpatient Rehabilitation Medicine Service at University of Washington Hospital for intensive communication intervention.

COMMUNICATION AUGMENTATION APPROACHES

Descriptions and Definitions

The following section contains descriptions and definitions of approaches and will serve as an introduction to the vocabulary used throughout this book. Readers are cautioned that in no way can it be considered a complete overview of augmentative or alternative approaches available. We have provided a list of more complete references at the end of this chapter (Schiefelbusch, 1980; Silverman, 1980; and Vanderheiden, 1978). The generic term "communication augmentation" refers to any approach designed to support, enhance, or augment the communication of individuals who are not independent, verbal communicators in all situations. Other terms used synonymously include assistive, alternative, nonvocal, or nonoral communication. Approaches to communication augmentation have been broadly classified as either *aided* or *unaided*.

Unaided Approaches

Unaided approaches are those that rely on gestural communication. As with any augmentative approach, selection decisions involve determining whether or not the individual's capabilites are commensurate with the requirements of the approach and whether or not the approach has the potential for meeting the user's communication needs. Gestural approaches vary along a number of dimensions, which have been described in detail by Peterson and Kirshner (1981) and Yorkston and Dowden (1984). Symbolic load refers to the extent to which a gesture is an arbitrary symbol for the concept it conveys. Some gestural approaches are highly symbolic, whereas others are more concrete. The symbolic load of a gestural system must be considered for a number of reasons.

Highly symbolic gestures may be difficult for the language impaired user to learn. However, concrete or referential gestural systems have limited potential to convey a wide range of messages. The motoric complexity of any gestural approach must also be considered. A single gesture may involve a fairly simple movement or entail a highly complex sequence of movements. Motoric complexity is an important consideration in selection of an augmentative approach because successful use of some gestural systems may be precluded by problems in motor learning and motor control. Gestural approaches may serve a number of communicative functions. Some replace speech, whereas others serve to facilitate or "deblock" verbal expression.

Aided Approaches

Aided approaches are those that depend on a system or device of some kind. These range from the "light" technology of traditional communication boards and books to the high technology of computer-based electronic communication systems. Although the variety of commercially available systems may initially be somewhat confusing, nearly all systems contain three basic components—control, process, and output. Each of these basic components will be discussed in turn.

System Control. Control of most systems has two aspects, display and interface. *Display* refers to what the user observes when operating the system. For example, the control display of a conventional typewriter is the keyboard with all selections displayed on the keys. A second type of display consists of a panel containing a number of light locations. The lights are illuminated to offer choices to the user. Symbols contained on the display may vary from standard orthography to a variety of alternative symbol systems for nonreaders. Some systems, such as that based on the Morse code and described in Chapters 3 and 7, do not require a control display. Users memorize the codes rather than having selections presented to them via a visual display.

An *interface* is the means by which the user actually controls the communication system. Interface control may involve single or multiple switches activated by displacement, touch, light intensity, or electromyographic (EMG) control. The selection of an interface for a communication augmentation system depends primarily upon the physical control of the user. Minimal physical control may require a single switch interface with a *scanning* control display, such as the ones described in Chapters 7 and 11. The user selects a communication option by activating the switch at the moment the selection is displayed. Users with greater control can direct a cursor to the desired location using multiple switches or a joystick. Still another type of interface option is called a *direct selection* interface. A conventional typewriter with its multiple switch, displacement interface is a familiar example of this control option.

System Process. The second basic component of communication augmentation systems will be referred to as *system process*, the function performed by the system. A variety of process options are represented in commercially available communication augmentation systems. Some systems only transmit the message without enhancing, storing, or decoding it. A conventional typewriter is such a system because the depression of a key corresponding to a letter of the alphabet results in the printing of that letter only.

A second type of process involves the retrieval of coded messages. These messages may be words, phrases, or sentences and may be called up by the selection and activation of a code. Communication augmentation systems that have message retrieval functions differ in degree of flexibility. Some are programmed at the factory and cannot be changed without modifying the hardware of the systems. Others can be preprogrammed by the manufacturer to meet the specific vocabulary needs of the nonspeaking individual. Other units are programmable in the field by the user, an attendant, or other adults who have knowledge of the particular system even without formal computer programming knowledge. The field programmable units offer the most flexibility because their vocabulary or selection options can be altered or enhanced at any time when new communication demands are placed on the user.

The third process found in many commercially available communication augmentation systems allows the individual to prepare a message, store it, and then retrieve it by activating a single "memory read" or "recall" choice. The chief benefit of this memory storage or message retrieval process is a saving in time for communication partners. Using such a system, nonspeaking individuals can take as much time as they need to prepare a message correctly; however, the message can then be delivered to the communication partner at a relatively rapid rate.

System Output. The third basic component of communication augmentation systems is the system *output*. Output choices available in communication augmentation systems can be divided into two broad categories—visual and auditory. Some visual and all auditory outputs are transient in nature. For example, the output of a communication board is visually transient, in that the communication partner observes as letters or words are indicated by the user, and no permanent record is left. Visual output systems, such as television screens and marquee-type displays, are semitransient in that the output is displayed only temporarily. Many communication augmentation systems, such as a typewriter, strip printer, or computer-driven printer, produce permanent visual output.

Numerous communication augmentation approaches have been designed to serve individuals with not only a wide variety of physical, linguistic, and cognitive capabilities but also diverse patterns of social, educational, and vocational communication needs. The number of commercially available systems has grown rapidly in the years since our center has been established. We have begun to rely heavily on the commercially available systems, often doing exhaustive searches for an appropriate commercial system before we even consider developing a one-of-a-kind system. This reliance on commercial systems has occurred for a number of reasons. First, we operate on a fee-for-service basis, and the simplest one-of-a-kind systems are extremely costly. Second, commercially available systems are increasingly flexible, reflecting an appreciation of individual needs and capabilities of nonspeaking clients. Third, the commercial vendors of communication augmentation equipment in the Seattle area have been extremely helpful in making systems available to us on a trial basis when necessary.

SELECTION DECISIONS

In 1977, when our center began selecting communication augmentation approaches for nonspeaking individuals, the number of potential choices was more limited than it is today. Even so, it quickly became apparent to us that the selection process could not be a simple trial-and-error one in which the clinician would run through the list of available alternatives until an acceptable approach was found. We began to realize that the same questions were arising time after time in our evaluations. For those questions that were routine, we began to develop standard assessment and selection approaches. The following is not an attempt to outline a theoretical model of system selection. Rather, it is a process that has developed as a consequence of our attempts to systematize our assessment protocols. Figure 1–1 illustrates our decision-making process when we are attempting to select an augmentative communication approach for a nonspeaking individual. It involves two parallel lines of questions that converge as the final decisions are being made.

Needs Assessment

The first line of questions reflects an attempt to specify the communication needs of the user. Needs assessment involves the identification of specific communication tasks which the nonspeaking individual must perform in order to function in particular environments. We have begun to rely heavily on the results of the needs assessment to set intervention goals. The goal of our intervention is almost never to normalize communication. Normal speech is so rapid, efficient, and versatile that it is simply out of the reach of nearly all of the nonspeaking individuals that we see. Because we are unable to aim for normalcy, the decision about goals becomes somewhat more difficult. As we work together we have begun to narrowly define our goals in terms of the communication needs of the individuals we serve. By answering the question, "What does this person need from the communication augmentation approaches?" , we are forced to create a list of specific statements that define and describe the goals of intervention.

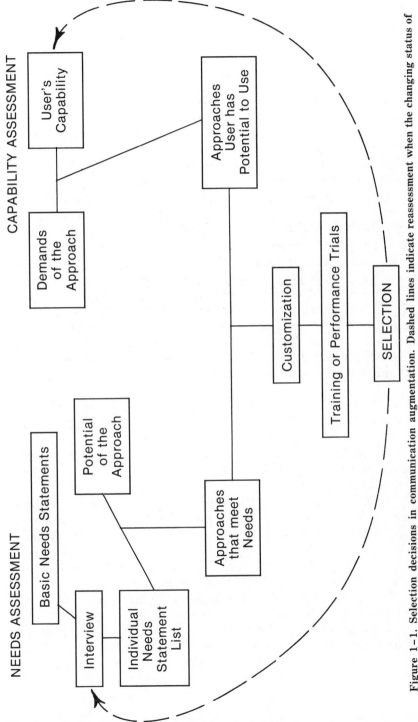

Figure 1-1. Selection decisions in communication augmentation. Dashed lines indicate reassessment when the changing status of the user brings about either a change in communication needs or a change in capability.

Needs Statements. Appendix I contains a basic list of needs statements that we are currently using. These statements are grouped into a number of categories. Some statements relate to the communication partners — e.g., Does this patient need to communicate with someone who cannot read? Some relate to the location or the patient's position — e.g., Does this patient need to communicate while lying supine, or while sitting in bed? Still other statements relate to the message needs — e.g., Does this person need to signal emergencies, to make a small number of medical care–related requests, to provide unique information?

You will see as you review the basic needs statements that many are quite general. However, others are more specific. We have found that different environments place certain specific demands on the user. For example, the school setting may demand that the nonspeaking student produce written material in a standard format (i.e., typed on an 8½ x 11 inch sheet of paper), to fill in responses on prepared worksheets, and to take part in group discussions. On the other hand, the intensive care unit environment may require the nonspeaking patient to communicate in the presence of oral intubation or intravenous lines. Thus, we have begun to individualize the list of needs statements for users and their communication environments. Among the most frequent environments are the acute medical or intensive care units (Chapters 7 and 9), schools (Chapters 10 to 15), residences (Chapter 10), and vocational settings (Chapters 3 and 12).

The Needs Assessment Interview. We carry out the needs assessment in an interview format. Our staff, together with the primary partners, family members, and the nonspeaking person, complete the questionnaire. As a starting point, a number of judgments are made about each needs statement on basic needs list. The questions we ask are roughly as follows:

1. Is the need currently being met satisfactorily by another approach? For example, the need to signal answers to yes or no questions is often met by head nods rather than by an augmentative device.

2. Is the need a mandatory one? If the answer is "yes," priority is given to finding a device that meets that need.

3. Is the need desirable but not mandatory? If the answer is "yes," a lower priority is given to meeting that need.

4. Is the need unimportant? If the answer is "yes," the need is no longer considered in system selection.

5. In the foreseeable future might this need become mandatory? This question is particularly important when selecting systems for

children who may have one set of communication needs for today and a much more complex set of needs for the future. We must have information about future need in order to make selections now that will lead to approaches appropriate for the future. Chapter 4 illustrates the case of a child with changing communication needs, which had to be considered in the system selection process.

The needs statements listed on the basic Needs Assessment Protocol often serve as a starting point. Any number of new needs may be added for those individuals who must function in environments where heavy communication demands are placed on them. Chapter 3 contains a description of a needs assessment for an individual in a vocational setting where a large number of unique needs were added to the basic list.

The interview format for the needs assessment serves a number of functions. It helps the nonspeaking person, the family, and important communication partners specify objective goals for the intervention. The process also allows the staff and those they serve to come to some kind of consensus about the goals of intervention. By detailing where, when, with whom, and for what purposes the systems are to be used, potential selection mistakes may be avoided. Early in our service program before we began to rely so heavily on needs assessment, we sometimes selected an approach only to find that it did not meet some specific but important communication needs for the user. For example, a system with only a printed output does not allow someone to interact effectively in a group. Or a system that can only be operated a few hours a day when the user is sitting in a wheelchair does not serve that individual's broad needs to have an accessible system throughout the day.

In short, the needs assessment serves several purposes. It encourages the staff and those they serve to develop specific, mutually agreed upon goals. Second, it encourages early consideration of how the system is to be used so that systems are selected with the greatest potential to meet the individuals' actual needs. Third, it acquaints the clients and their communication partners with communication possibilities that they may have not considered.

Decision Making Based on Communication Needs. When the needs assessment interview is completed, our staff has a list of specific statements that detail what the augmentative communication approach must allow the use to do. We also estimate future communication needs. The next step in the selection process is to match this needs list with the systems that are available. From a practical point of view, using the needs assessment as a foundation for the selection process also allows the evaluation team to eliminate from consideration approaches that clearly do not meet the specific needs of the nonspeaking individual, even though that individual may have the capability to use the approach. This reduces the number of options that must be considered and simplifies what has become an extremely complex decision-making process.

Assessment of User Capability

Deciding on an augmentative communication approach involves two parallel lines of questioning. As outlined in the previous section, the goal during the needs assessment phase is to identify the approaches that have the potential to provide the functions that the user requires. Our goal for the user capability assessment is to identify the approaches that nonspeaking persons are able to use successfully. Thus, the capability assessment involves gathering enough information to decide whether or not the nonspeaking individual has the potential to use particular augmentative communication approaches.

A Criterion-Based Assessment. Our assessment strategy can be described as a criterion-based rather than an exhaustive assessment. A clinician using the exhaustive assessment strategy would ask, "What is the maximum level of performance on a series of cognitive, language, motor, or visual tasks?" In the criterion-based assessment, the clinician asks, "Is the level of performance on a series of cognitive, language, motor, or visual tasks suffcient to allow the individual to use a given approach?"

Our preference for the criterion-based approach is based at least in part on practical considerations. For example, when performing a capability assessment in the intensive care unit, where time is at a premium because of the patient's fragile medical condition, we are not interested in maximum levels of performance (e.g., knowing that the patient spells at the ninth or the tenth grade level). Rather, we are interested in knowing whether or not he or she possesses the "threshold" of abilities to use the particular augmentative approach. Therefore, we sample minimal levels of performance on a particular skill. If a typing system has the potential to meet the patient's communication needs, we will sample spelling on simple tasks, perhaps asking the patient to spell words which we predict would be part of the vocabulary used in the environment. This vocabulary may be at the third or fourth grade level.

System Requirements. Our criterion-based capability assessment requires both formal and an informal assessment of cognition, language, motor control, and vision. Candidacy for use of any approach depends on its cognitive and linguistic requirements. Some of the more basic approaches require only elementary understanding of communication intent and the cause-and-effect relationship that exists between the selection of a message and the communicative consequence of that selection. For example, the user needs to know that there is a relationship between activation of the switch, sounding of a buzzer, and getting the attention of those in the vicinity. Other systems are extremely demanding cognitively and linguistically. They require high-level performance on spelling, language formulation, and learning tasks.

Formal Testing. The formal assessment of language and cognition in an individual with severely limited response options and experience is often a difficult and time-consuming one. To date, tests with multiple-choice response formats have been popular for the evaluation of nonspeaking individuals, because response can be made by pointing, eye-gaze, or a yes or no indication to the choices presented by the examiner. Examples of such tests include the Peabody Picture Vocabulary Test (Dunn, 1965), Raven's Progressive Matrices (Raven, 1960), Test of Auditory Comprehension of Language (Carrow, 1973), Gates-MacGinitie Reading Test (Gates and MacGinitie, 1965, 1969), and the spelling and reading subtests from the Peabody Individual Achievement Test (Dunn and Markwardt, 1970).

For nonspeaking individuals who come to our center for outpatient evaluations, as much as possible of the formal testing is done by the referring agency before we see the client. Appendix II contains our Outpatient Intake Form. This form asks for extensive information about cognitive, language, reading, and spelling abilities. Knowing this information at the time of our intake evaluation is useful to us in a number of ways. First, often the referring agency knows the nonspeaking client much better than our staff. They have the luxury of conducting their testing in short segments over an extended period of time. Second, having preliminary cognitive and language information also allows our staff to focus our assessment on a small number of potentially appropriate alternatives.

At best, formal assessment of nonspeaking individuals is inexact and must be supplemented by extensive observation of performance in daily situations in order to make a valid decision about the candidacy of a user for a particular augmentative approach. Relying on the experience and expertise of the referring agency allows us the get a glimpse into how the nonspeaking individual functions in natural settings as well as in a formal testing situation.

Selecting Control Options. Perhaps the most critical step in the selection of augmentative communication approaches is the choice of control options. Without a reliable control approach involving both a display and an interface, even the most elaborate of systems cannot be used effectively. As with the cognitive and language testing, we use a criterion-based approach to the assessment on a nonspeaking individual's capacity to use certain control options.

Displays are selected in order to compensate for whatever vision problems might be present. Often this can be accomplished by using large displays or taking special care to position the display with the visual field of the user in mind. When more severe visual problems are present, auditory displays may be necessary. This approach was necessary for two cases described in Chapter 10. In general, we do not test vision with exhaustive assessments of visual acuity, visual scanning, and tracking skills or tests of visual fields. Rather, we use the display of the particular system in the assessment. The questions to our neuro-ophthalmologist specifically relate to the potential visual deficits which may interfere with use of that system.

The selection of a reliable interface is often the most challenging portion of the entire selection process, especially with individuals with severe motor control problems. With such individuals, the team must often develop proper seating and head control or support before interface selection can be considered. Chapters 2, 4, 5, and 10 describe cases in which complex decisions were required for interface selection. For individuals possessing more extensive motor control, several interface options may be available. If this is the case, interface selection may be secondary to other considerations.

During the past several years, the staff at the Center has explored two general approaches to motor assessment. Initially, we began with exhaustive approach. We attempted to assess all potential movement patterns that might be employed in interface control, including the hand, arms, head, feet, and legs. After the exhaustive assessment was completed, we selected the sites and interface approaches to be explored in more detail. In time, we gradually reduced our motor assessment even for individuals who could physically tolerate extensive assessment. The exhaustive approach was time-consuming and therefore expensive. We realized that, as our experience in the communication augmentation field increased, we were not using much of the information derived from the exhaustive approach. For example, we have found "direct selection" systems to be far superior to "scanning" systems in terms of the potential for maximizing communication rate. Therefore, when motor control assessment revealed the capability for direct selection, we did not need to pursue the motor assessment related to single switch control. Of course, if motor control for direct selection was marginal, we would assess further to determine if other control sites and control options would be more efficient.

In time, our motor assessment became criterion-based, as we realized that a limited number of control options are usually utilized in the communcation augmentation field. These types include direct selection with many switch choices, four switch control with a joy stick or four separate switches, two switch control, or single switch control. Our initial motor assessment is now designed to identify the control type and the anatomic site(s) that offer the potential for accurate, efficient interface control. During the initial motor control screening, we observe our clients as they perform a specific switch control task. The task is a simple one, which assesses the user's ability to activate, release, and reactivate control options. The examiner counts at a metered pace, and the client is asked to activate the switch at a given count, to release it one or two counts later, and to reactivate it still later. This task allows the examiner to observe not only rate and accuracy of switch activation and release but also the effects of anticipation. Knowledge of a client's ability to accomplish each phase of motor control is essential to the selection of an interface.

In addition, a number of other factors are involved in the choice of interface control options. First, the social acceptability of the control to a client and the family requires careful attention. For example, in Chapter 10 we describe a tongue control interface which was socially acceptable to our client but would undoubtedly be unacceptable to others. Second, the movements associated with interface control, especially for clients with cerebral palsy, are an important factor in final interface approach. For example, some clients demonstrate excessive abnormal reflexes and associated movements when controlling an interface with the hand. However, the same individuals may demonstrate a marked reduction in associated movements while operating a head-controlled interface. Third, the interface approach should be minimally fatiguing to the client. Chapter 7 describes the communication system operated by a man with amyotrophic lateral sclerosis (ALS), who demonstrated the motor control for a head-mounted direct selection interface. However, our assessment of fatigue revealed his inability to use this approach for long periods of time, and therefore we selected a brow switch, which could be operated while the head and neck could be supported. Fourth, the impact of posture on interface control is vital aspect of motor assessment. If the communication needs assessment reveals that the communication system must be operated in several postures — in the wheelchair, in bed, or on the couch — motor control should be assessed in these positions.

The posture of some clients does not permit accurate, efficient interface control. Prior to completion of the motor assessment an intervention program to eliminate or reduce postural limitations may need to be completed. This program often involves selection of an appropriate seating system.

At the conclusion of an initial capacity assessment, we attempt to select the interface control approach(es) that appears to be available to a client and to predict the communication system(s) that can be controlled with it. We also have reviewed the cognitive, linguistic, and visual capabilities, identifying communication approaches that are compatible with them. By this time, we have also completed the communication needs assessment, which identifies the functions that must be performed by the communication approach. With this basic understanding of capabilities and needs, we make our initial selection of approaches and arrange for performance trials and training to clarify our choices. Finally, funding options are explored to support equipment purchase and training when necessary. Reviewing the 12 cases presented in the casebook, we found that funding came from a number of different sources, including legal settlements, Division of Vocational Rehabilitation, school districts, medical insurance, Washington State Public Assistance, and private funds.

Performance Trials

Performance trials are the last phase of the system selection process shown in Figure 1–1. Before approaches are finalized, we give the nonspeaking individual the opportunity to use the system. Performance trials for adults typically proceed through a number of steps. The approach selected as a result of the combination of the needs and user capacity assessment is first customized to reflect the motor control, visual, and vocabulary needs of the user. The nonspeaking individual, family, and other important communication partners are instructed. The use and care of the equipment, including troubleshooting of minor problems and battery recharging schedules, are reviewed.

Control Drills. The remainder of the intervention focuses on training the individual to use the approach. We begin this training with what we call "control drill." As the word "drill" implies, these exercises focus on learning the approach rather than on communication per se. For example, if an electronic system with a four switch directed scanning control was selected, the control drills would involve having the nonspeaking individual use the control switches to activate selected locations on the display board. Progress could be measured by counting the decreasing number of switch activation errors. Another simple means of monitoring improvement is to measure the time required to activate ten preselected locations accurately. When you measure total time, errors are reflected in increases in time required to achieve accuracy. For children, timed drills alone may not be appropriate. Rather, children may need to learn switch control via activation of toys during play. In the case of both children and adults, the goal of control drills is to achieve accuracy in operation of the approach while placing minimal communication demands on the user.

Once accuracy is achieved at slow rates, the goal of the control drills is to increase the rate. We often spend considerable time in training accuracy. It has been our experience that relatively high accuracy is required in order to avoid frustration, especially if the user is attempting to communicate urgent messages. At best, the output rates that communication augmentation systems allow are slow. Any reduction in accuracy magnifies the slow rates by extending the self-correction time. By spending enough time on control drills to ensure accurate perforance, levels of frustration can be reduced. Once accuracy is achieved, increased rate becomes important. However, we have found that accuracy cannot be sacrificed for a faster rate without causing problems.

Control drills facilitate what our staff calls "motor learning." We distinguish it from the conceptual learning that also needs to take place during training in use of a communication augmentation approach. Learning that you activate a location by holding a light sensor over the location for a given period of time, that you can correct an error by activating the "delete" location, or that you produce a typed printout by activating the "printer" location are examples of conceptual learning. Many of the nonspeaking adults we see can learn the concepts needed to operate a communication augmentation system after only a brief period of instruction. Motor learning, on the other hand, requires hundreds and perhaps thousands of repetitions of a particular movement pattern before that pattern becomes so automatic that the user can execute it with consistent accuracy and very little concentration on the movement task itself. The learning of consistent motor patterns is essential to the successful operation of many communication augmentation approaches.

Message Preparation Tasks. The next phase of performance trials involves message preparation. Such preparation tasks are designed to simulate communication more closely than the control drills we have just described. However, these tasks do not require interaction with a communication partner. The clinician asks the nonspeaking individual to produce a series of known messages using whatever communication augmentation approach has been selected for that individual. Messages of various types, lengths, and formats are prepared and analyzed for accuracy, rate, level of independence, and the user's endurance. In short, message preparation tasks can be considered "communication to dictation." Materials are selected to reflect the capabilites and communication augmentation approach used by the nonspeaking individual. Generally, however, a series of words or phrases are dictated to the nonspeaking individual, who is asked to repeat them as rapidly and accurately as possible using a particular communication augmentation approach.

When evaluating nonspeaking persons who are "new" to a particular approach, message preparation tasks can be used to estimate the potential for increased rate that may come with learning. We do this by performing what we call "cued" versus "uncued" dictation trials. The uncued portion of this trial is similar to the message preparation task just described. In it, the nonspeaking individual is asked to communicate the dictated message as accurately and as rapidly as possible but is given no help. During the cued task, the clinician assists the user in some way. This assistance may take the form of identifying the location of a particular letter on an unfamiliar keyboard arrangement or providing the code under which a particular message is stored. The differences between cued and uncued performance give a rough indication of the increases in communication rate that will come about as the user becomes more familiar with the system.

During the final stages of message preparation training, we encourage our nonspeaking users to prepare communicative messages, such as writing letters or preparing memos to individuals who are not present. We have found this to be a good transition between dictation tasks and conversational communication interaction. It gives the user the opportunity to practice with a functional communication task. Yet a letter-writing or memo preparation task is not nearly as demanding in terms of speed, accuracy, and flexibility is as conversation. In effect, this communication task gives the user all the time needed to prepare a message and to check for and correct errors.

Training in Interaction.   During the last phase of performance trials, we work with interactive rather than message preparation tasks. Interaction tasks are designed to simulate natural communication situations in which information is exchanged between communication partners. Interaction tasks require the nonspeaking individual to transmit a message to a communication partner who does not have prior knowledge of the specific message being conveyed. The communication partner has the opportunity to confirm the content of the message or to ask any questions to clarify messages that are not completely understood. Interactive tasks offer the possibility of quantifying communication breakdowns and breakdown resolution strategies as well as quantifying the accuracy and rate of message preparation. They also provide a format for assessment of one of the most important dimensions of the communicative use of augmentation systems — conversational control. The term "control," when used in this sense, refers to the communicator's ability to manage or direct the interaction. It represents a broad range of behaviors that occur in communicative interaction, including obtaining and maintaining turns, initiating exchanges, responding to a partner's initiation, interrupting a partner's turn, and changing roles from responder to initiator. It has been our experience that one of the consequences of the slow message preparation rate is difficulty controlling communication interactions. Therefore, training of both the system user and the important communication parters is often necessary to prevent interaction from becoming a simple, one-sided question and response sequence.

We have begun to assess and train interaction using simple direction giving tasks. In such a task, a nonspeaking adult sees a card with a number of geometric shapes of varying colors, sizes, and locations on it. The interaction is structured so that the communication partner can not see the card. In the instructions, the nonspeaking individual is asked to give directions to the partner, so that the partner can reproduce the figure on a blank sheet of paper. The pair is free to interact in any way they wish. The communication partner may ask confirmatory questions or do whatever is needed to complete the task. Each turn can be coded for a number of control related factors.

PLANNING FOR THE FUTURE

The portion of this chapter on selection decision has been a general one and can be considered to illustrate the management plan for users of communication augmentation systems. It captures the selection of the most appropriate approach for a moment in time. Of course, the picture becomes much more complex when attempting to serve an individual whose situation is not stable or for whom change is expected. This lack of stability is the usual situation with two large populations of nonspeaking individuals — all children and those adults with progressive conditions. With these populations, our staff must attempt to make educated guesses about the future. We attempt to make at least two types of predictions. The first concerns future needs; the second, future capabilities. These glimpses at the future are extremely important for the management of nonspeaking persons. For adults with progressive conditions, the prediction allows the selection of an approach that will serve their communication needs for the longest possible time (see Chapters 7 and 8 for descriptions of cases which a degenerative disease is present). For children, the predictions dictate the educational direction that would prepare the child for future use of increasingly more effective communication approaches; see Chapter 4 for an illustration of such a case. With nonspeaking individuals whose situations are not stable, both the needs assessment and the assessment of capability must be repeated periodically in order to confirm the appropriateness of the current approach, to modify it, or to replace it with another approach.

REFERENCES

Carrow, E. *Test of auditory comprehension of language.* Austin, TX.: Learning Concepts, 1973.

Dunn, L. M. *Expanded manual for the Peabody Picture Vocabulary Test.* Circle Pines, MN.: American Guidance Service, 1965.

Dunn, L. M., and Markwardt, F. C. *Peabody Individual Achievement Test.* Circle Pines, MN.: American Guidance Service, 1970.

Gates, A. I., and MacGinitie, W. H. *Gates-MacGinitie Reading Test.* New York: Teacher's College Press, Columbia University, 1965, 1969.

Peterson, L., and Kirshner, H. Gestural impairment and gestural ability in aphasia: A review. *Brain and Language,* 1981, *14,* 333–348.

Raven, J. C. *Guide to the standard progressive matrices.* London: H. K. Lewis, 1960.

Schiefelbusch, R. (Ed.). *Nonspeech language and communication: Analysis and intervention.* Baltimore: University Park Press, 1980.

Silverman, F. L. *Communication for the speechless.* Englewood Cliffs, N.J.: Prentice Hall, 1980.

Vanderheiden, G. *Non-vocal communication resource book.* Baltimore: University Park Press, 1978.

Yorkston, K. M., and Dowden, P. A. Nonspeech language and communication systems. In A. Holland (Ed.), *Language disorders in adults.* San Diego: College-Hill Press, 1984.

ADDITIONAL READINGS

Albert, C. Procedures for determining the optimal nonspeech mode with the autistic child. In R. L. Schiefelbusch, (Ed.), *Nonspeech language and communication: Analysis and intervention.* Baltimore: University Park Press, 1980.

American Speech and Hearing Association. Position statement on nonspeech communication. *ASHA,* 1981, *23,* 577–581.

Beukelman, D. R., and Yorkston, K. M. Nonvocal communication: Performance evaluation. *Archives of Physical Medicine and Rehabilitation,* 1980, *61,* 272–275.

Beukelman, D. R., Yorkston, K. M., Gorhoff, S. C., Mitsuda, P. M., and Kenyon, V. T. Canon Communicator use by adults: A retrospective study. *Journal of Speech and Hearing Disorders,* 1981, *46,* 374–378.

Carlson, F. *Alternative methods of communication.* Danville, IL: Interstate Printers and Publishers, 1982.

Cohen, C. G., and Shane, H. C. An overview of augmentative communication. In N. J. Lass, L. V. McReynolds, J. L. Northern, and D. E. Yoder (Eds.), *Speech, language, and hearing.* Philadelphia: W. B. Saunders, 1982.

Coleman, C. L., Cook, A. M., and Meyers, L. S. Assessing the non-oral clients for assistive communication devices. *Journal of Speech and Hearing Disorders,* 1980, *45,* 515–526.

Fristoe, M., and Lloyd, L. L. A survey of the use of non-speech communication systems with the severely communication impaired. *Mental Retardation,* 1978, *16,* 99–103.

Harris, D., and Vanderheiden, G. C. Augmentative communication techniques. In R. L. Schiefelbusch, (Ed.) *Nonspeech language and communication: Analysis and intervention.* Baltimore: University Park Press, 1980.

Kraat, A., and Sitver, H. *Features of commercially available communication aids.* Shreve, OH: Prentke Romich Co., 1983.

Musselwhite, C. R., and St. Louis, K. W. *Communication programming for the severely handicapped: Vocal and non-vocal strategies.* San Diego: College-Hill Press, 1982.

Schiefelbusch, R. L. (Ed.). *Nonspeech language and communication: Analysis and intervention.* Baltimore: University Park Press, 1980.

Shane, H. C. Early decision making in augmentative communication use. In R. L.Schiefelbusch, and D. Bricker, (Eds.), *Early language: Acquisition and intervention.* Baltimore: University Park Press, 1980.

Shane, H. C., and Bashir, A. S. Election criteria for the adoption of an augmentative communication system: Preliminary considerations. *Journal of Speech and Hearing Disorders,* 1980, *45,* 408–414.

Shane, H. C., and Cohen, C. A discussion of communication strategies and patterns by nonspeaking persons. *Speech, Language and Hearing Services in Schools,* 1981, *12,* 205–210.

Silverman, F. H. *Communication for the speechless.* Englewood Cliffs, NJ: Prentice-Hall, 1979.

Vanderheiden, G. C., and Grilley, K. (Eds.). *Nonvocal communication techniques and aids for the severely physically handicapped.* Baltimore: University Park Press, 1976.

Vanderheiden, G. C., and Harris-Vanderhieden, D. Communication techniques and aids for the nonverbal severely handicapped. In Lloyd, L. L. (Ed.), *Communication assessment and intervention strategies.* Baltimore: University Park Press, 1976.

Vickers, B. (Ed.). *Non-oral communication system project 1964–73.* Iowa City: The University of Iowa, 1974.

Yoder, D., and Kraat, A. Intervention issues in nonspeech communication. In J. Miller, D. Yoder, and R. L. Schiefelbusch (Eds.), *Contemporary issues in language intervention.* ASHA Report, #12, 1983.

CHAPTER 2

Ruby

Etiology: Brain-stem hemorrhage
Onset: 44 years of age
Approach: Express I
Focus: This chapter presents the case of a woman who suffered a brain-stem hemorrhage that resulted in severe motor impairment but intact cognitive and language skills. Of interest is the sequence of selection and training in the use of an optical headpointer to operate the Express I as both a communication and a wheelchair drive system. Limitations of the system for conversational interaction are discussed.

BACKGROUND

Ruby arrived at our center four months after a brain-stem hemorrhage associated with a chiropractic manipulation. A 44 year old active mother of three teenagers, she had worked as a dental assistant and managed a small farm prior to injury. Following the injury, she underwent intubation and required ventilatory assistance for a brief period. Her left diaphragm remained paralyzed. A gastrostomy was performed because of severe swallowing problems that led to aspiration pneumonia prior to admission for rehabilitation. Because she was unable to move her legs and arms voluntarily, she required extensive nursing care. Initially she controlled only eye and forehead movements. Her inability to speak made her dependent on others.

INITIAL EVALUATION

Early Communication System

Upon her arrival to the Rehabilitation Unit, Ruby communicated by answering yes or no questions and by using a dependent scanning approach. She signaled "no" by closing her eyes and "yes" by leaving them open and raising her eyebrows slightly. The dependent scanning approach involved a small (8½ by 11 inch) chalkboard with the letters of the alphabet listed vertically along the lateral margins — A through L on the left margin and M through Z on the right. As communication partners pointed to each column sequentially, Ruby raised her eyebrows to signal the appropriate column. The partner then scanned down the column until Ruby signaled the desired letter. The partner wrote the message letter by letter in the center of the board. Partners familiar with Ruby's frequent messages would often attempt to increase communication rate by guessing the completion of messages. Ruby confirmed the accuracy of the guesses by responding with a "yes" or "no" signal. Through these approaches Ruby communicated basic self-care, health care, and interpersonal information to those who understood the system and who would take the time to communicate with her.

Communication Needs Assessment

The needs assessment was completed by Ruby, her primary nurse, and a speech-language pathologist. During this assessment, Ruby indicated her extreme frustration with the current communication approach. She wished to have a system that would allow her to produce an unlimited number of unique messages independently. She did not consider preprogrammed words or phrases mandatory. She wished to be able to use the system both in bed and while in a wheelchair. Despite the fact that all of the requirements identified in the needs assessment were general, we did not seek to make the list more detailed at this point because it was sufficient to give us a general direction for the first phase our intervention. Namely, Ruby needed to control a system reliably and independently. This would allow her to produce messages in a letter-by-letter fashion.

Capability Assessment

Motor control.   When Ruby was admitted to the Rehabilitation Unit, she was quadriplegic and had control of only eye and forehead movements. She exhibited little neck movement and was unable to hold her head up while sitting but could move her head laterally when supine. During the course of hospitalization, some isolated biceps and finger flexion movements returned, but these were minimal and they could not be used functionally. Ruby's ability to maintain an upright head posture while seated improved gradually during the course of her hospitalization. She achieved limited control of head movements and could rotate her head from side to side but had little neck flexion. Endurance on tasks that required head control improved steadily.

Speech. Motor control for speech was severely impaired. Ruby was unable to produce phonation, or to achieve lip closure, while supine. Motor control abilities for speech improved slightly but did not reach a functional level. She was able to achieve lip closure at a rate of one closure per second. This is extremely slow in comparison to normal movement rates. She was able to elevate the tip of her tongue slowly. Tongue control was sufficient to allow her to produce four or five vowels understandably. Another factor limiting her potential for functional speech appeared to be respiratory and phonatory control. Ruby's left diaphragm remained paralyzed. She also was unable to generate sufficient breath pressure to produce phonation voluntarily. Ruby was able to produce a voice only when lying supine. Even in this optimal position, however, she succeeded in producing a voice in only 70% of her attempts. She continued to practice speech throughout the course of her hospitalization. At the time of discharge, there were approximately 10 words she could use functionally, but only when lying down and only with listeners who had become familiar with her speech. This word list included mom, up, hi, bye, no, and yeah.

Language. Extensive language testing was difficult to complete initially because of her limited speech, the slowness of the alphabet spelling system, and problems with fatigue. However, language skills appeared to be adequate for an augmentative approach that relied on spelling. She was able to answer even the most rapidly presented yes or no questions accurately and without delay and to spell messages using the alphabet spelling system without error. Spontaneous spelling skills (spelling to dictation) were assessed using the Wide Range Achievement Test (Jastak and Jastak, 1965). Performance on this test placed her at the 8.1 Grade Level. Vocabulary recognition, as measured by the Peabody Picture Vocabulary Test (Dunn, 1965), was over the 18 year old ceiling of the test. No word finding problems were evident in conversational interaction with Ruby.

Vision. Visual acuity was unchanged since the injury. Ruby wore no corrective glasses, but complained of double vision at times, when she was fatigued. She was able to read typed material, magazines, and newspaper print without difficulty. The neuropsychologic assessment revealed some mild visual perceptual problems.

Cognition. Only limited neuropsychologic testing was performed because of Ruby's motor deficits and lack of understandable speech. The Categories Test from the Halsted-Reitan Battery (Halsted, 1947; Reitan and Davidson, 1974) was administered because it required only multiple choice selection. This early testing indicated that Ruby's abstract conceptual thinking was just below the normal cut-off level.

INTERVENTION

Interface Selection

The Options. Following the completion of the needs and capability assessments, an intervention program was begun while Ruby was an inpatient on the Rehabilitation Unit. She participated in daily physical therapy, occupational therapy, and speech treatment sessions. The first question to be answered was whether Ruby had the motor control and endurance to access a large direct selection control display with a headlight pointer, or whether she would need to use a scanning approach with one or two switches. The direct selection approach would be preferable because of its potential for faster communication rates than with the scanning approach.

The Headlight Pointer. Ruby was fitted with a headlight pointer mounted on a headband and positioned over her right ear. With this she indicated the letter choices on the alphabet chalkboard described earlier. Instead of scanning the board, Ruby's partners now confirmed the letter indicated by Ruby. Initially, Ruby was only able to approximate the letter locations. As she practiced, her accuracy increased. She began to use the headlight pointer for sentence-length messages. Use of the headlight pointer increased Ruby's communication rate. Because her partners would hold the alphabet spelling board, Ruby could use the system in a variety of locations and positions. She used it in bed, lying either supine or on her side, and in her wheelchair, seated either upright or reclined. For most partners, communication using the headlight pointer was approximately three times faster than the scanning system. However, the system required set-up in that the light needed to be positioned on Ruby's head and the direction of the beam adjusted. This process took less than 30 seconds, but many partners found short messages more conveniently communicated with the totally dependent scanning system.

Training Neck Strength and Control. A physical therapy program was begun to improve the strength and motor control of Ruby's neck muscles. By this time in her rehabilitation, a manual wheelchair had been customized for her with appropriate trunk and head support. This allowed her to sit upright for short periods of time. Once she was able to sit throughout the half hour speech treatment session, Ruby began a motor training program utilizing the Express I communication system.

The Express I Communication Aid. This is a portable microprocessor-based electronic communication system that may be operated in either a direct selection or a scanning mode (Fig. 2–1). The direct selection display panel contains 128 locations. In the standard system, Levels 2, 3, and 4 can be programmed with letters, words, or phrases by the user. The Express I has a correctable visual display that can be viewed by the user during production of messages; messages can also be printed on a strip of thermosensitive paper tape.

The Optical Headpointer. The Express I can be controlled by a number of switches or interface options. In order to take advantage of Ruby's head control, the optical headpointer was selected for a trial. When the optical headpointer is directed toward the desired location, a "beep" indicates that the selection has been accepted and the corresponding character or word(s) will appear on the visual display. The lag time between selection of a location and its acceptance can be varied. This means that the sensor can sweep across a number of locations but the selection is accepted only when the user stops at the desired location for a predetermined period of time.

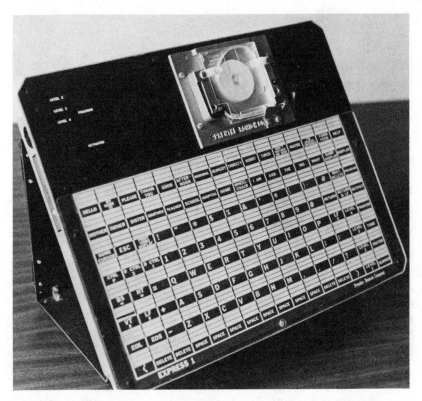

Figure 2–1. Express I communication aid with direct selection overlay.

Motor Training Drills.   Ruby could operate the Express I with the optical headpointer mounted much as the headlight pointer had been (Fig. 2-2). During this phase of her program, Ruby was to select locations on the display panel as a motor training task without attempting to communicate. These drills had a number of purposes. The first was to increase the speed and accuracy of her selections within the area of the board, which was roughly equivalent to the size of her alphabet spelling board. The second was to increase the area on the board that she could accurately access. In order to take advantage of the entire 128 locations, both head stability and range of motion to direct the light sensor to the perimeter of the display needed to be improved. During this motor training drill phase of her program, Ruby used the system only when sitting. The snap-on stand was used to position the system nearly vertically. The Express I was then positioned on a hospital table, adjusted to the appropriate height, and moved close to the patient.

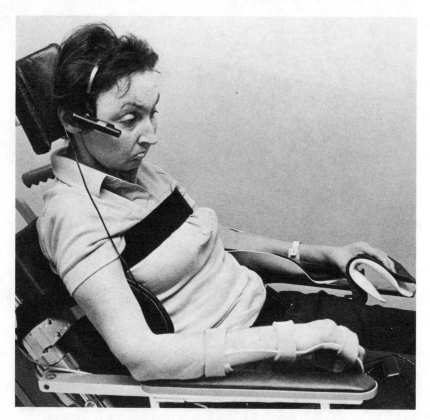

Figure 2-2. The optical headpointer used to access the Express I.

Continuous Versus Intermittent Feedback. Ruby had some difficulty making the transition from the headlight pointer to the optical headpointer. Although the mounting and movement requirements for the two interfaces are nearly identical, the two operate quite differently. The headlight pointer provides continuous feedback. The beam of light is continuously visible on the display surface so that the user knows at all times where the pointer is being directed. The optical headpointer, on the other hand, provides only intermittent feedback. Because it is a light sensor rather than a light beam, the user knows where the pointer is being directed only when the light is activating at a particular location on the display. When the pointer is either between locations on the board or off the display panel entirely, the user receives no feedback. Not knowing specifically where her optical headpointer was directed was particularly troublesome for Ruby when she was attempting to activate locations close to the edges of the board. Whenever she directed the optical headpointer "off the edge" of the display, she had no feedback about how far from the edge it was. Our makeshift solution to this problem was to tape the headlight pointer and the optical headpointer together on the same headband. This was not an ideal solution because the two pointers could not easily be aligned to point at exactly the same location. However, Ruby accommodated to these slight differences and found the feedback provided by the light beam to be useful in these early motor training drills. Once accuracy began to improve, she found that she no long needed the continuous visual feedback. Readers should be aware that Ruby's training occurred in 1982. Since that time, a dual pointer has become available commercially through Prentke Romich Company. With this instrument, both light beam and light sensor can be directed at identical locations on the display panel.

Monitoring Progress. Ruby's progress was monitored during this phase of intervention with a single word dictation task. Once a week she was asked to spell a number of short words randomly selected from a large list. Words were dictated one at a time. Ruby was allowed to correct any errors by selecting a "delete" function, then retyping the letter. Error corrections increased the time required for message preparation. We measured the total time needed to type the words accurately. The time decreased from over 7 minutes (0.7 word/minute) to less than 1 minute (5 words/minute) during the course of training.

Initial Communicative Uses. Once Ruby's accuracy improved to the point that she was making few errors, she began to use the Express I as a communication system. Initially, the system was accessible to her only during the two or three hours of the day in which she was sitting in her wheelchair. Therefore, the first communicative uses involved Ruby's writing letters to be sent to family and friends. Ruby's accurate operation of the system and use of it for a communicative function marked the end of our first phase of intervention.

Mounting the System

During the first phase of intervention, the primary question was whether Ruby's motor control would allow her to use a direct selection rather than the slower scanning approach to operate the Express I communication system. After approximately six weeks of training, we were satisfied that she would be able to operate the system using the optical headpointer, a headband mounted light sensor. The second phase of intervention involved mounting the system so that Ruby would have access to it in a number of situations. Funding for this and other equipment was provided through a legal settlement.

Disposition Plans.   Roughly at the beginning of the second phase of intervention, Ruby's disposition began to be discussed. At the end of her rehabilitation, she would be discharged to a nursing home in a small community about 300 miles from our center. The questions that faced the team at this point revolved around what equipment she would need in order to maximize her ability to function independently there.

Specific Needs Statement.   A second needs assessment, much more detailed than the first, was completed by the team in cooperation with Ruby and her family. At this time, specifics of system use could be described along with details of how the communication system could be integrated into her other mobility and environmental control systems. Although the general needs were unchanged since the the first needs assessment, a number of more specific statements were added to the original list (Table 2–1). This list of specific need statements was drawn from the larger pool, which appears in Appendix I. Ruby wished to use the system both in bed and while sitting in her wheelchair. She wished to have the system with her as she moved from place to place in her electric wheelchair. This required that the system be mounted on the wheelchair rather than placed on a stationary table. Because she relied on busy staff or perhaps on staff not thoroughly familiar with her system, ease of movement of the system from wheelchair to bed and vice versa was mandatory. Nursing staff also felt that the system must be easy to position out of the way during transfers. Ruby wished to switch independently from communication to wheelchair drive and back again. She wished to be independent in preparing unique messages.

Table 2-1. Specific Needs Statements for Ruby

Positioning
　In bed:
　　I,M　While supine
　　D　　While lying on side
　　I,M　While sitting in bed
　Related to mobility:
　　M　　In an electric wheelchair
　　D　　While the chair is reclined
　　M　　Arm troughs
　Other needs related to positioning:
　　M　　Easy transfer from wheelchair to bed

Communication Partners
　　D　　Someone who cannot read (e.g., child or non-reader)
　　D　　Someone with no familiarity with the system
　　D　　Someone who has poor vision
　　D　　Someone who has limited time or patience
　　D　　Someone who is across the room or in another room
　　D　　Someone who is not independently mobile
　　D　　Several people at a time
　　D　　Someone who is hearing impaired

Locations
　　I,M　In multiple rooms with the same building
　　M　　In dimly lit rooms
　　M　　In bright rooms
　　D　　Outdoors
　　D　　While moving from place to place within a building
　　M　　In more than two locations in a day

Message Needs
　　I,M　Call attention
　　I,M　Signal emergencies
　　G　　Answer yes or no questions
　　I,M　Provide unique information
　　I,M　Make requests
　　M　　Carry on a conversation
　　M　　Express emotion
　　I,M　Give opinions
　　I,M　Convey basic medical needs
　　M　　Greet people
　　I,M　Prepare messages in advance

Modality of Communication
　　I,M　Prepare printed messages
　　D　　Prepare auditory messages
　　D　　Talk on the phone
　　I,M　Communicate with other equipment, e.g., environment control
　　　　　units
　　D　　Communicate privately with some partners
　　D　　Via formal letters or reports

Key:
　M　=　Mandatory
　D　=　Desirable but not mandatory
　I　=　Independence is required on this task
　G　=　Gestures were used to meet this need

She continued to feel that preprogrammed messages were desirable but not mandatory. She indicated that she had all the time she needed to prepare messages in a letter-by-letter fashion. A review of Table 2–1 also indicates that Ruby considered a number of other needs, including speech output, to be desirable but not mandatory.

Wheelchair Driving. Because so many of her communication needs also related to the mobility system, the question of how Ruby was to drive her wheelchair was the next major decision. A number of wheelchair control options were considered. Some were ruled out almost immediately. The first was a sip-and-puff control of the Du-It wheelchair. Ruby did not have sufficient lip strength or quickness to use this interface reliably. A hand-controlled joystick was ruled out because the minimal finger flexion that had returned was not sufficient to control the wheelchair reliably.

Joystick Control. A collar-mounted, chin-controlled joystick was the first option that Ruby could reliably use; a collar-mounted joystick is illustrated in Figure 2–3. Although she had the motor control to use this interface when it was appropriately positioned, a number of problems became apparent once trial use was begun. The first problem was Ruby's inability to move the joystick out of the way during episodes of coughing. When she was operating the wheelchair, the rubber cup attached to the joystick was positioned firmly under her chin. Ruby continued to experience severe swallowing problems with occasional episodes of choking, during which her head would be thrown forward. When this occurred during practice sessions, clinicians would simply move the joystick out of the way. If a coughing episode were to occur when Ruby was alone, however, she would have no easy way of moving the joystick to allow forward movement of her chin. Her continuing swallowing disorder also caused another problem with respect to use of the joystick interface. She was unable to swallow saliva consistently. Although the extent of drooling varied from day to day, moisture occasionally would seep into the mechanism of the joystick. Placing plastic covering over the joystick to protect it against moisture damage reduced Ruby's control.

Wheelchair Control Via the Express I. Because of the many drawbacks experienced while using the chin-controlled joystick, another interface was sought. Through the efforts of Prentke Romich Company, Rehab Equipment Services of Seattle, and our program, the Express I was factory-programmed with a fifth level, which was used as a wheelchair control system. Thus, Ruby could use the optical headpointer not only to operate the communication system but also to operate the

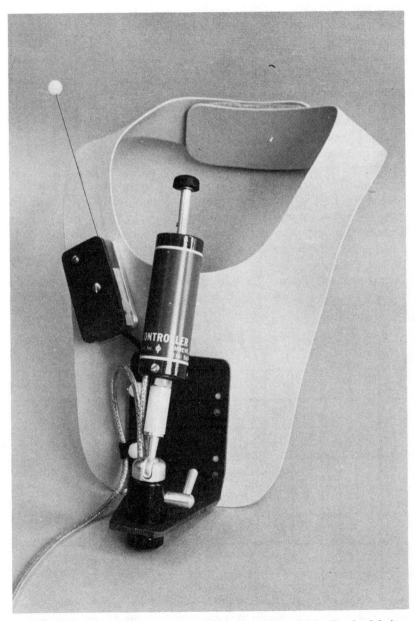

Figure 2–3. The collar-mounted joystick control for the Du-It wheelchair.

electric wheelchair. Figure 2–4 illustrates of the display panel as it functions when the fifth level of the Express I is activated. This level allows Ruby to control three functions or channels on the Du-It electric wheelchair by activating the area designated "W/C" (wheelchair) and then "DU-IT SCAN" for the scan function. In Channel 1 of the Du-It system, the direction squares for driving are activated. The center location of the driving square is "neutral." Moving up from neutral directs the chair forward; moving down from neutral directs the chair in reverse. Activation of the locations to left or right of neutral directs the chair in sharp turns, whereas diagonals to left and right direct the chair in gradual turns. In Channel 2 of the Du-It system, Ruby could set the speed of the wheelchair at either low, medium, or high speeds. The final channel of the Du-It system allows Ruby to recline the back of the wheelchair so that she can obtain pressure relief without being transferred back to bed. The two columns to the far left of the wheelchair operation level (Level 5) were programmed to cancel the wheelchair function and return immediately to Level 1 of the communication system. Thus, in the case of an emergency or a problem in controlling the wheelchair, Ruby could make one sweeping head movement to the left and stop the wheelchair at once.

Mounting the System.   The mounting of the Express I for use as a wheelchair control system required greater system stability than would

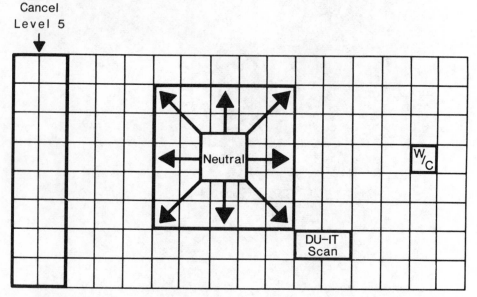

Figure 2–4. A schematic illustration of Level 5 of the Express I used for wheelchair control.

have been necessary if it were to serve solely as a communication system. In this application, Ruby was required to operate the system while the chair was moving. Mounting was accomplished with an aluminum mounting block and rod manufactured by Prentke Romich Company. This rod is attached to the Express I via a customized plate. Figure 2–5 illustrates the system positioned ready for communication, and Figure 2–6 illustrates the system swung away in the position used during transfers. The system could be swung away, for transfers without having to disconnect any of the electric connectors.

Mounting the Express I on the hospital bed was accomplished by positioning the wheelchair near the bed, lifting the system with the mounting plate and rod from the wheelchair's mounting block, and inserting the rod into a similar block on the bed (Fig. 2–7).

More training. When Ruby used the Express I for communication, she had became accustomed to a position almost directly in front of her line of vision. However, when she began wheelchair trials using the system, an unrestricted line of vision for wheelchair maneuvers became mandatory. Thus, the entire system had to be lowered and tilted slightly so that Ruby could see over the top of it. The new slanted position initially meant the target locations were more difficult for Ruby to access. However, she soon became accustomed to the new position. Similar systems are being developed by Prentke Romich with see-through display panels for wheelchair drive.

Control for Communication Versus Wheelchair Drive. Two problems became apparent when Ruby attempted to drive the chair using the optical headpointer. The first was the slight movement of the Express I as the wheelchair started and stopped, turned, or went over rough ground. As a communication system, the Express I can be placed on any sturdy table or wheelchair lapboard. However, when used as a wheelchair driving system, the issue of stability was of real concern in the mounting. Stability was increased by adding a second support strut so that both sides of the system were firmly attached to the body of the wheelchair. During transfers this second strut was simply detached first and swung out of the way.

The second problem that arose when Ruby began to drive the wheelchair was related more basically to the way in which she controlled the system. Use of the optical headpointer to control the communication system had by this time become an easy motor control task for Ruby. She used head movement and changes in head positions to direct the optical headpointer to the desired locations on the display panel. She did so quickly and almost without error. When first beginning to use

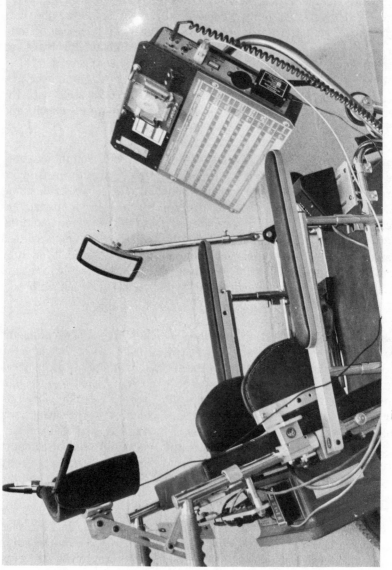

Figure 2–5. The Express I mounted on a wheelchair.

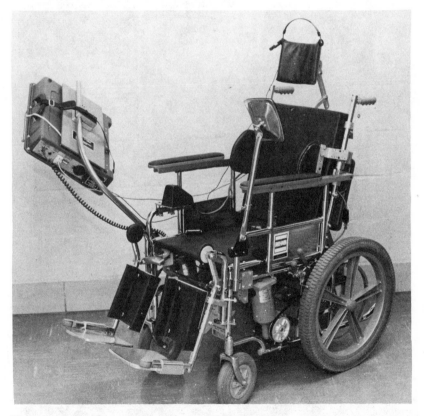

Figure 2–6. The Express I mounted on a wheelchair and swung away in a position ready for subject's transfer.

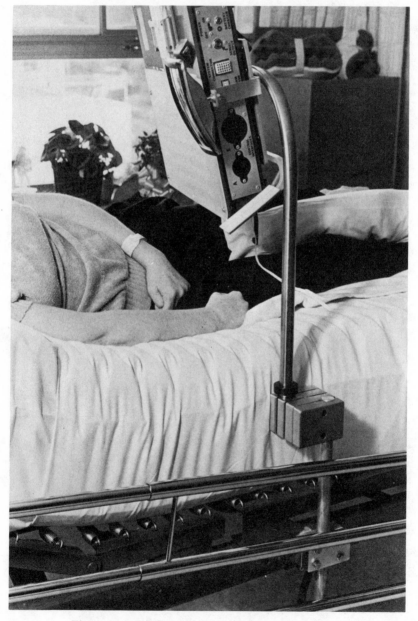

Figure 2–7. The Express I mounted on a hospital bed.

this wheelchair interface, Ruby had a natural tendency to use these same head movements to scan her visual field to see where she was going. Because the head must remain steady to direct the optical headpointer at the appropriate locations, Ruby learned to scan the environment with eye movements while using head movements only to direct the light sensor. From the perspective of motor control training, we were fortunate that Ruby had had approximately two months of practice with the communication system before she attempted the wheelchair drive. The wheelchair drive is a more difficult task than communication. The consequences of error when controlling the communication system are only as serious as the time lost in going back to correct the mistake. Errors in wheelchair driving have the potential of being much more serious. Although completely unplanned, the sequence of training to proficiency on the communication system before attempting the wheelchair drive system turned out to the correct training sequence.

Transition to the Nursing Home. The final weeks of her inpatient hospitalization involved preparing Ruby for the move to the nursing home. In our center, the staff had been familiar with the system from its inception. In the nursing home the staff had probably never seen such a complex system before. We attempted to make this transition as smooth as possible in a number of ways. First Ruby was instructed in all aspects of both the communication and the mobility systems. She was taught to do as much as possible independently. For example, with the communication system, she could change the acceptance speeds, turn the printer on or off, and program and delete entries in Levels 2, 3, and 4. For those functions she was unable to perform independently, she learned to give instructions so that others could do them. For example, she took responsibility for instructing her caregivers about battery charging and instructing the staff to change the paper cassette before it ran out.

An indexed notebook with a brief description of the operation of all the equipment was prepared by our occupational therapist. This notebook contained information about how the systems were to be set up and maintained. It contained numerous photographs of details from connecting power cables to recharging batteries and changing the thermo tape cassettes. It also contained a list of phone numbers and mailing addresses if a problem should arise with any of the systems. Finally, when a representative of the vendor of Ruby's equipment delivered the equipment to the nursing home, he conducted an "in-service" demonstration for about 30 staff members.

RUBY'S COMMENTS

As we began to prepare this chapter, we contacted Ruby to ask her permission to use her story and to obtain her comments about her communication system. Both she and her family reported that she uses the system extensively, at times using a cassette of paper in one day. She commented that she had improved her typing rate since leaving the hospital. During our conversation, her typing rate was 12 words/minute, more than double the rate she had been achieving the last time we had measured it. As our discussion proceeded, it became apparent to me how much Ruby depended on the system. She wrote, "When it works, it's great! When it doesn't it's a point of frustration. It almost seems it chooses to be down when I really want it." Ruby went on to tell me that her children were able to visit her only one day during the Christmas holidays. Because the system had not been recharged properly the night before, she was left with only her alphabet chalkboard for their visit.

Many of the problems she reported related to the extensive demands she places on the system. For example, she mentioned that her message tapes frequently become so long that she runs over them as she operates her wheelchair. She has had a basket attached to the system to catch the lengths of paper tape she produces.

Some subtle but important changes in Ruby's motor control had occurred in the year since discharge. When she left our rehabilitation center, she was fed through a gastrostomy and had occasional episodes of choking when she was unable to handle her saliva adequately. When she returned, she was meeting all of her nutritional needs orally. Episodes of drooling and choking had also decreased. These changes, along with slight improvement in head and neck control, made it possible for Ruby to drive her wheelchair with the chin-controlled joystick. She found this wheelchair control option especially useful when driving outdoors in the bright sunlight because the light-sensor interface of the Express I was not always reliable.

Her only major concern about the function of the Express I communication system related to its lack of "speech." (The speech module was not yet available when Ruby's system was initially purchased.) Ruby stated, "I didn't realize what a good idea speech would be. I find it next to impossible to get people to read the tapes and even when they do look at the tape, they don't read closely enough. I also have a blind friend I would spend time with if the system could talk." We are currently seeking funding for the purchase of an Express III system with speech for Ruby.

QUESTIONS FOR THE CLINICIAN

Question 1. Ruby's intervention was complex and technically sophisticated. How was decision-making managed to reduce conflict among professionals serving her mobility, self-care, and communication needs?

The decisions described in this chapter were made over an 8 month period in which Ruby was hospitalized as an inpatient on our Rehabilitation Unit. One key to the minimal conflict that occurred on the team was the sequential nature of the decisions. In other words, our questions were "small" and asked in an appropriate order. We did not forced ourselves to answer big questions too early. If at our first team meeting after we had initially evaluated Ruby the team had been required to list the equipment that she would eventually require, the debate would have gone on for hours without satisfactory resolution. We did not have the information to answer such global questions during the first months of rehabilitation. Instead we asked a much smaller question, "What type of interface could Ruby control?" Even this question could not be answered until Ruby was fitted with a wheelchair with adquate trunk and head support and given a period of training on the interface options. Once the control interface had been selected, the specific communication, mobility, and environmental control systems could be selected. Once the Express I had been selected for communication and mobility, decisions could be made about mounting it for maximum function in the nursing home environment.

As you read a chapter that condenses months of small decisions in a few pages, there is a tendency to think that all the decisions were made at once or that the final destination had been in sight all along. This was not the case with Ruby and indeed may not be the case with many nonspeaking individuals who need periods of training before selection questions can be answered and the next step in the decision-making process made. Like the situation with many other nonspeaking individuals, selection decisions for Ruby involved months of training, customization, and trial use.

Question 2. Why was the first phase of the needs assessment such a general one?

The needs assessment is designed to identify specific requirements of the commmunication approach for the environment in which it will be used. Early in Ruby's rehabilitation we could not easily predict these needs because we had little information about disposition. The injury had been recent, and return of motor function would have drastically affected her communication needs. Finally, the general needs identified in our first needs assessment were sufficient to give us focus for the next several months: namely, to find a reliable means by which Ruby could control a system and prepare messages in a letter-by-letter fashion.

Question 3.   You indicated that Ruby used her communication system primarily for memo preparation rather than interpersonal communication. Why was that the case? What changes could be made to increase interpersonal communication for Ruby? What communication aid characteristics encourage interpersonal communication?

Ruby's case was clearly successful in that a woman with severe physical deficits was able to perform a number of important functions independently. In reviewing this case, however, it is also easy to find areas in which the technical capability and the training failed to provide adequate levels of function. In terms of communication, this area is the potential for normal conversational interaction.

Perhaps another phase of intervention should have been added to the first phase, in which a system was selected, and the second phase, in which it was mounted. The third phase of intervention would focus on maximizing interaction skills. When she left the rehabilitation center, Ruby was able to operate the Express I as both a communication and a mobility system. She did so essentially without error. However, the pattern of communication could still be described as "memo preparation." When alone she would prepare long letters to those outside of the hospital and memos to those around her. She used the system infrequently in face-to-face conversation. Ruby did not or could not easily take part in this important type of communication for a number of reasons. In closing this case presentation, we will list some of these reasons and offer some potential technical and nontechnical solutions.

The first barrier to conversational interaction was the fact that Ruby's partners typically did not face her during communication because they could not easily see the display as she prepared messages. Partners either had to wait until the entire message had been prepared and printed out or stand behind the wheelchair and lean over to see the display. More recent systems offer at least a partial solution to this problem in that some allow displays that are clearly visible to both communication partners.

The second barrier to normal conversational interaction was the fact that Ruby was unable to switch from one communicative message preparation task to another. As was indicated earlier, her style was to write long memos and letters. Often we would find Ruby spending her free time in the day room creating a memo to someone not present. If we wanted to have a brief conversation with her, she would have to stop "midstream" in her text preparation. If the system had two memories, Ruby could switch back and forth between them when interrupted. She could store her partially completed letter in one memory and use the second memory for conversation. After finishing the conversation, she could return to the first memory and resume her letter writing.

Finally, both the rate of message preparation (maximum of 12 words/minute) and the output mode (printed output only) interfered with the potential for interaction. Recently a research project has been completed at our center (Farrier, Yorkston, Marriner, and Beukelman, submitted for publication). In the project, we compared conversational control of nonimpaired adults when they spoke versus when they were restricted to the use of a communication augmentation system. Results suggested that the limited communication rate and timing of message presentation that were imposed by communication augmentation systems severely restricted subjects' ability to maintain conversational control. Subjects who maintained conversational control did so only if they sacrificed communication efficiency.

Although her motor control deficits limited her selection rate, other strategies for enhancing conversational control might have been explored. For example, locations could have been programmed with words or entire phrase in an effort to increase the overall communication rate. Ruby was never particularly interested in programming self-care messages in Levels 2, 3, and 4 so that they could be printed quickly. The pressure to increase the rate of message preparation was not urgent for Ruby because she did not use the system in an interactive manner. Ruby always felt that she had plenty of time to prepare any desired messages in her free time. However, the slowness of message preparation clearly interfered with conversation. The preprogramming of a number of "conversational devices" may have facilitated interaction.

Question 4. Have you had experience with other individuals in situations similar to Ruby's for whom the interaction issues were managed more effectively?

Yes, as we completed this book, we were serving Dee, another woman with a brain-stem hemorrhage. Dee had been a rehabilitation patient in our center in 1978. At the time of her discharge, her motor control capabilities were very similar to Ruby's. Dee communicated using two approaches. First, she used a dependent scanning approach similar to the one described in Chapter 10. She blinked her eyes to signal "yes" as her communication partner spoke the alphabet to her. Second, she typed her messages using a Canon Communicator, which she activated with a customized mouth wand (Fig. 2–8). Although this system was slow and cumbersome, Dee was able to write letters, leave notes, and prepare comments to guide conversations with visitors. There were several limitations to this approach. She was unable to communicate in bed with the Canon system. Second, the Canon had to be positioned precisely for Dee to access all of the keys with the mouth wand. Third, the mouth wand encouraged excess drooling. Finally, the Canon Communicator had several limitations as a conversational tool. The listener had to rip off the tape on which the message was printed in order to read it. Communication was limited to "listeners" who could read. The Canon did not provide an effective way to communicate conversational control messages. However, even with all of the shortcomings of this approach, Dee was able to express herself at a rate of 10 words/minute. At the time the system was provided for her, we were hopeful that it would be replaced with an approach that would meet more of her communication needs.

When the Express I system became commercially available, we gave Dee a trial with it. She demonstrated the ability to access the system using an optical headpointer. An effort to obtain funding was begun. Due to a variety of health and funding related issues, responses to funding requests were delayed. By the time funding was approved, the Express III system with speech synthesis and Minspeak software had become commercially available and was purchased for her. Dee controlled the system with optical headpointer just as Ruby had. Messages could be prepared in a letter-by-letter fashion or retrieved in their entirety using the Minspeak mode, described below. Output could be printed or spoken via the "text-to-speech" algorithm in the system.

The Minspeak option provides a method for addressing the messages that are stored in a communication system. Figure 2–9 shows a number of line-drawing symbols. Each of the symbols represents a concept or several concepts. With Minspeak, the user selects a message to be stored in the memory of the communication system for retrieval at another time. The message is retrieved by selecting the sequence of symbols associated with the message. For example, the symbols: "?," "Wanted" poster, and "apple" might be used to signify the message "When do you want to eat?" The symbol sequence: "stop sign," "eye," and "telephone" might mean "Please wait until I am finished speaking." The relationship between the symbol sequence and the message they

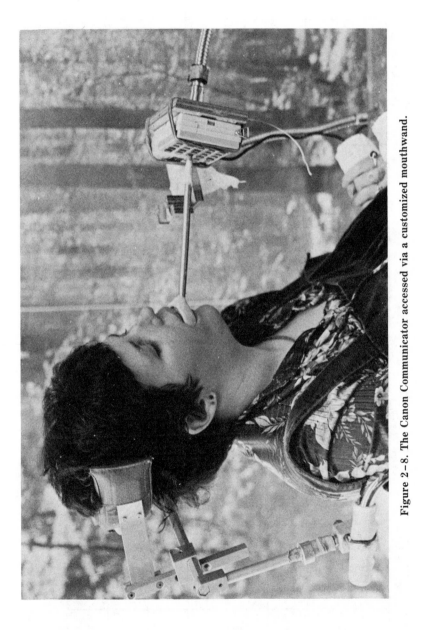

Figure 2–8. The Canon Communicator accessed via a customized mouthwand.

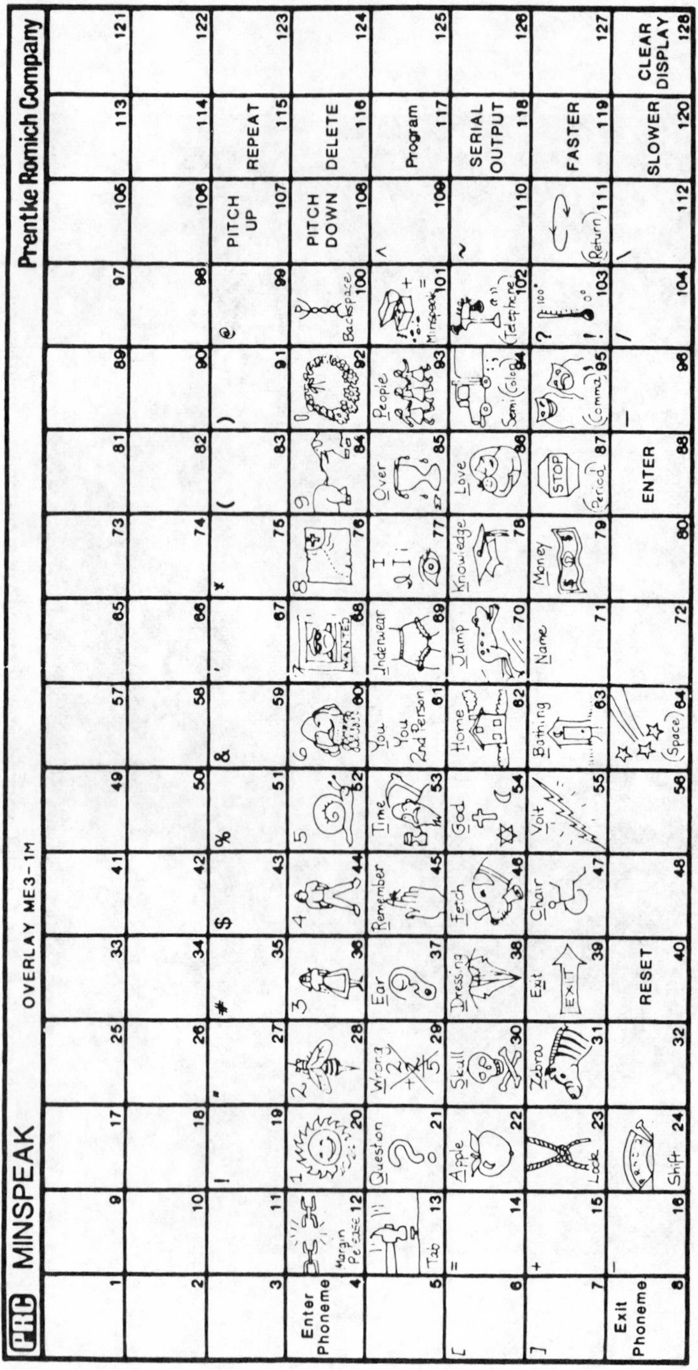

Figure 2–9. The Minspeak display panel.

represent is arbitrary and is determined by the user and those who serve as their consultants. All of the Minspeak programming can be completed in the field. A large number of words, phrases, and sentences can be stored in the system.

Dee's training with the Express III system with Minspeak was completed in several stages. First, she learned the operation of the system using a letter-by-letter spelling approach. During this phase she practiced the motor control necessary to access the system accurately and efficiently. After two weeks of use, she was able to formulate a message at a letter-by-letter "typing" rate of 12 words/minute. During this phase, Dee and her two primary attendants listed the messages that they expected Dee would be interested in retrieving in a hurry. Their initial list is as follows:

1. I would like a drink, please.
2. Please change me.
3. I have heartburn.
4. I have a headache.
5. Please move me back in my chair.
6. Move my left foot.
7. Scratch my nose, please.
8. I'm hungry. How about a snack.
9. Please call my folks for me. Tell them . . .
10. Could you bring in the radio and find something good.

A review of this list reveals the absence of conversational control phrases. Dee had not spoken for six years. She no longer used conversational "grabbers" to control interactions. To the original list, we added the following messages.

1. Tell me more.
2. I don't understand.
3. I didn't hear you. Say it again.
4. You don't say.
5. Uh-huh.
6. I'm not finished yet.
7. Could I talk to you a minute.
8. Let me try that again.

After the initial list of messages was compiled, Dee and a speech-language pathologist from our center began to develop strategies to select symbol sequences to address each message. The initial symbol in a sequence usually represented the action or activity of the message. For example, all requests and desires were represented by the "Wanted" poster, all eating and drinking were represented by the "apple," all questioning was represented by the "?," all telling of messages to another person was represented by the "telephone," and all greetings and conversational control activities were represented by the "lei." The second symbol was usually assigned to the person(s) involved in the message. The concept "I" was implied. "You" was represented by the printed word "you." Individual names were represented by the location on the Minspeak display containing the first letter of the name. The third and fourth symbols were selected by Dee to assist her in individualizing the symbol sequence for a particular message.

As messages were programmed, Dee's attendant and the speech-language pathologist recorded the symbol sequence and the messages in a dictionary. If Dee forgot a symbol sequence, we were able to assist her. Also in case of a system failure, we would have a complete record to be used in reprogramming the system.

At the time this chapter was written, Dee was using the Express system for all communication. She was able to type at a rate of 15 words inute. She had programmed 50 messages and was able to use approximately 90% of them in conversational communication. The rapid retrieval of messages through Minspeak was used frequently; however, Dee preferred to spell most of her messages letter by letter, as this mode allowed the careful formulation of messages to express her ideas accurately. The speech mode is used with increasing frequency as Dee learns to manage her interpersonal communication in a more natural manner than was permitted with her previous communication approaches.

One obvious frustration remains. Dee spends much of her time writing letters and preparating printed material for persons prior to their visits with her. When she is the middle of text preparation, she is reluctant to engage in conversational activities because she must first print or clear the portion of the message in the marquee display before conversing through speech. Dee reports that she would prefer a "second memory," so that the text preparation could be interrupted and held in one memory as she converses with someone using the second memory. At the conclusion of the conversation, she could return to the first memory and continue the text preparation where she had left off.

ACKNOWLEDGMENTS

In cases such as Ruby's or Dee's, which extend over months or years and involve a large number of health care professionals, many people are deserving of our thanks. In Ruby's case, the first of these are Ruby and her family, who tolerated the apparent slowness of the decision making process and the fact that the equipment never seemed to work perfectly the first time. Next, thanks must go the the entire health care team, to Suzanne Wilson, OTR, who created the discharge notebook, to Jan Lambert, RPT, who worked on wheelchair drive with the optical headpointer, and to Nancy Lowe, Speech Pathology Intern, who did much of the early work in motor control training with the Express I. Sharon Benham, RN, Ruby's nurse, and Diana Cardenas, MD, attending physician, wrote many letters requesting just 10 days more of funding for extended rehabilitation. Marvin Sorderquist of the Engineering Applications Program at University of Washington and Dean Iverson of Rehab Equipment Service provided much of the technical expertise that made all the equipment work together.

Dee's intervention was long-term, and so many individuals were involved that we cannot remember them all. In particular we would like to thank Marvin Soderquist for his work on Dee's initial system. Ken Frye of Rehab Equipment was particularly supportive during the Minspeak application. A special thanks goes to Nancy Zytkowitz and Doris McCann for their day-to-day assistance with the system.

REFERENCES

Dunn, L. M. *Expanded manual for the Peabody Picture Vocabulary Test*. Circle Pines, MN: American Guidance Service, 1965.

Farrier, L., Yorkston, K. M., Marriner, N., and Beukelman, D. R. Conversational control in non-impaired speakers using an augmentative communication system. Submitted for publication.

Halsted, W. C. *Brain and language*. Chicago: University of Chicago Press, 1947.

Jastak, J. F., and Jastak, S. R. *The Wide Range Achievement Test manual*. Wilmington, DE: Guidance Associates, 1965.

Reitan, R. M., and Davidson, L. A. *Clinical neuropsychology: current status and application*. New York: Winston/Wiley, 1974.

ADDITIONAL READINGS

Baker, B. Minspeak. *Byte*, 1982, *7*, 186–203.

Beukelman, D. R., and Poblette, M. Maximizing communication rates of row-column scanning communication augmentation systems. A paper presented at the American Speech, Language, and Hearing Association Convention, Los Angeles, 1981.

Beukelman, D. R., and Yorkston, K. M. A series of communication options for individuals with brain stem lesions. *Archives of Physical Medicine and Rehabilitation*, 1978, *59*, 337–342.

Beukelman, D. R., and Yorkston, K. Communication interaction of adult communication augmentation system use. *Topics in Language Disorders*, 1982, *2*(2), 39–54.

Beukelman, D. R., and Yorkston, K. M. Computer enhancement of message formulation and presentation for communication augmentation system users. *Seminars in Speech and Language*, 1984, *5*(1), 1–10.

Beukelman, D. R., and Yorkston, K. Nonvocal communication: Performance evaluation. *Archives of Physical Medicine and Rehabilitation,* 1980, *61,* 272–275.

Beukelman, D. R., Yorkston, K. M., Gorhoff, S., Mitsuda, P., and Kenyon, T. V. Canon Communicator use by adults: A retrospective study. *Journal of Speech and Hearing Disorders,* 1981, *46,* 374–378.

Buzolich, M. Interaction analysis of augmented and normal adult communicators. Unpublished dissertation, University of California, San Francisco, 1983.

Calculator, S., and Dollaghan, C. The use of communication boards in a residential setting: An evaluation. *Journal of Speech and Hearing Disorders,* 1982, *47*(3), 281–287.

Calculator, S., and Lucko, C. Evaluating the effectiveness of a communication board training program. *Journal of Speech and Hearing Disorders,* 1983, *48*(2), 185–191.

Carlson, F. A format for selecting vocabulary for the nonspeaking child. *Language, Speech And Hearing Services in Schools,* 1981, *12,* 240–245.

Farrier, L., Yorkston, K. M., Marriner, N., and Beukelman, D.R. Conversation control in non-impaired speakers using an augmentative communication system. Submitted for publication.

Goodenough-Trepagnier, C., and Prather, P. Communication systems for the nonvocal based on frequent phoneme sequences. *Journal of Speech and Hearing Disorders,* 1981, *24,* 322–329.

Goodenough-Trepagnier, C., and Rosen, M. J. Model for a computer-based procedure to prescribe optimal "keyboards." Presented at the 4th Annual Conference on Rehabilitation Engineering, Washington, DC, 1981.

Harris, D. Communicative interactive processes involving nonvocal physically handicapped children. *Topics in Language Disorders,* 1982, *2*(2), 21–38.

Harris, D., and Vanderheiden, G. C. Enhancing the development of communicative interaction. In R. L. Schiefelbusch (Ed.), *Nonspeech language and communication: Analysis and intervention.* Baltimore: University Park Press, 1980.

Yoder, D. E., and Kraat, A. Intervention issues in nonspeech communication. In J. Miller, D. E. Yoder, and R. L. Schiefelbusch (Eds.), *Contemporary issues in language intervention.* ASHA Report #12, 1983.

CHAPTER 3

KEITH

Etiology: Spinal cord injury, cervical level 4 (C4)
Onset: 25 years of age
Approach: IBM-PC, with customized keyboard emulator
Focus: This chapter presents the case of a spinal cord–injured civil engineer who spoke normally but needed an augmentative writing system in order to return to work. Various typing systems available to individuals without good hand control are described. Keith was trained to use a Morse code–based keyboard emulator to operate an IBM-PC, which was the centerpiece for a technologically sophisticated workspace.

BACKGROUND

Keith is a 25 year old civil engineer who suffered a complete lesion at the fourth cervical vertebra in a motorcycle accident on 4/24/82. He was initially treated at another medical center, then transferred to Harborview Medical Center approximately 8 weeks after the accident.

Prior to his accident, Keith was employed in middle management of a local civil engineering firm. His job description included compiling and reporting on information obtained in the field regarding soil stability for the construction of high-rise buildings in downtown Seattle. This required him to communicate frequently with engineers and technicians in the field by telephone, by reports, or in person. He also compiled field reports, analyzed soil samples, and drew diagrams, maps, and charts. Other job-related activities included examining information available on multi-user data base computers in this region and writing summaries of findings for commercial customers. Immediately prior to Keith's accident, he was involved in the company's plan to computerize all of their data analyses; Keith was programming in *FORTRAN* to accomplish this change. The company had recently purchased a Cromemco computer and was working closely with a major computer service of the Northwest.

INITIAL EVALUATION

Communication Needs Assessment

On 6/25/82, Keith was referred to our service and to occupational therapy to evaluate his potential for a writing system. Decisions regarding a writing system for Keith depended first and foremost on a thorough assessment of his communication needs. After establishing his needs for writing, for telephone usage, and for computer communication, we could begin to determine the system or systems that could best meet these needs. Once potential systems were selected, we could undertake both training and the search for funding for this equipment.

Keith's communication needs could be specified in great detail because both the environment and the tasks required of him on the job were known. While in his office, his job required the following actions:

1. Communicate by telephone with colleagues in the office and in the field as well as with commercial customers in the Pacific Northwest.
2. Operate the Cromemco computer.
3. Transfer information from the Cromemco computer via a telephone modem to mainframe computers in the region.
4. Write formal reports summarizing the findings of the field engineers.
5. Write business letters.
6. Switch from one task to another—for example, make a phone call while writing a report, or check data in the computer while writing a letter.
7. Make and refer to calculations regarding soil analyses.
8. Take notes while reading or analyzing soil samples or during meetings, phone calls, or conversations.
9. Read and refer to reports by field technicians or engineers as well as texts and journals in the profession.
10. Draw or make changes in existing diagrams of sites, making notations regarding soil conditions.
11. Proofread and edit reports from other engineers or technicians.
12. Compile and refer to lists of phone numbers, addresses, references, ideas, plans, and so forth.

While in other locations within his office building, Keith's job required the following abilities:
1. Receive and make phone calls.

2. Refer to and make changes in analyses of soil samples in the laboratory.
3. Take notes during conversations, meetings, phone calls in all areas of the building, and while analyzing samples in the laboratory.
4. Make notes to himself or others as reminders or for information.

If he were confined to home at times, Keith's needs would be as follows:

1. Write and edit letters and manuscripts from the office.
2. Refer to and edit texts, manuscripts, or analyses on the Cromemco computer.
3. Make phone calls to colleagues who are on site or at the office.
4. Conduct business meetings by means of conference calls.

At other locations outside of his office or home, Keith's job involved the following requirments:

1. Make and receive phone calls.
2. Attend meetings and conferences.
3. Take notes during conversations, meetings, phone calls, conferences, and lectures.

After these needs were established, we contacted a variety of professionals in computer-related fields to help in the development of systems to meet Keith's needs. The consultants included a vocational counselor, a computer programmer who specializes in adapting computers for the handicapped, a computer software analyst, an employee at Keith's company responsible for the transition to the Cromemco computer, and two employees of the computer division of a major corporation, who volunteered their services. After this group completed most of the groundwork, a rehabilitation engineer was asked to make additional recommendations.

Capability Assessment

Motor Control. The motor control assessment was straightforward in that Keith's spinal cord lesion was complete at the level of the fourth cervical vertebra. Keith had lost all motor and sensory function below his shoulders; all functions above that level were intact. Keith's speech intelligibility was normal, with no deficits in articulation or resonance. The loss of function of the expiratory musculature as well as unilateral paresis of the diaphragm resulted in reduced respiratory support and decreased vocal volume. However, he spoke loudly enough for group and telephone conversation. While Keith had no impairment of the muscles of his face, his head control was impaired owing to the loss of innervation to the neck and shoulder muscles. He fatigued easily in any activities that required fine motor control of the head and neck.

Language and Cognition. Keith's spelling skills were assessed by means of the Wide Range Achievement Test (Jastak and Jastak, 1975) and determined to be at approximately the tenth grade level. Because there was no evidence of any cognitive deficits, this was presumed to be Keith's premorbid spelling level, and it was considered adequate for his position professionally.

From the needs assessment it was clear that Keith required a flexible computer-based system. While the consultants were researching the types of systems available that could meet Keith's needs, we assessed the control interfaces by which he could operate such a system. It was clear that Keith's motor impairments precluded the possibility of conventional typing on a keyboard. In general, there are several interface options available to most quadriplegic individuals:

1. Headwand for direct selection on the keyboard.
2. Mouthwand for similar direct selection.
3. Optical headpointer mounted on a headband for direct selection on a specially designed keyboard emulator.
4. Chin-controlled joystick for directed scanning control of a keyboard emulator.
5. Sip-and-puff controlled Morse code system via a keyboard emulator.
6. Speech recognition system in which the user speaks "commands" that are recognized by the computer.

At the time of the initial evaluation, it was not possible to assess the relative efficiency of all of these approaches for Keith. To evaluate the feasibility of speech recognition, we needed to rely heavily on the recommendations of the consultants described earlier. In addition, we could not compare Morse code to any system without training Keith in the basics of the system to know his potential proficiency level. However, it was possible to rule out approaches 1 through 4 as being potentially too fatiguing for an 8-hour work day. In addition, the Morse code and the speech recognition approaches were generally considered faster and more efficient than the directed scanning approach with the joystick. For these reasons, the team decided that the first step of the intervention phase would be to train Keith in the rudiments of Morse code. At the same time, the consultants were given the task of researching potential speech recognition systems and computer systems in general that might meet Keith's needs.

INTERVENTION

Learning the Codes

The Training Unit. Morse code training began on a modified A-Tronix Morse code translator (Fig. 3–1). This system, accessed via a sip-and-puff pneumatic switch, allows the user to print letters or numbers on a marquee display. When users "sip," creating negative oral air pressure, the keyer produces the "dahs"; when they "puff," creating positive pressure, the keyer produces the "dits." The switch is so sensitive that proficient users rely on their buccal muscles or subtle tongue movements to change oral air pressure for activation. Thus, a proficient user is able to breathe through the nose while continually generating code. Because the device contains an automatic keyer, the user does not need to sip twice to get two "dahs" within a letter, but only maintain that slight negative pressure continuously while the keyer emits a series of "dahs." The speed at which the modified keyer produces these automatically can be varied from approximately 2 to 20 words/minute, depending on the user's motor proficiency.

Training Sequence. There were three goals in the early stages of training. First, Keith had to learn Morse code. We relied on a system of visual mnemonics developed by Basic Telecommunications Corporation in Fort Collins, Colorado. This Morse Code Visual Display pairs the code graphically with the letter or number it represents. For

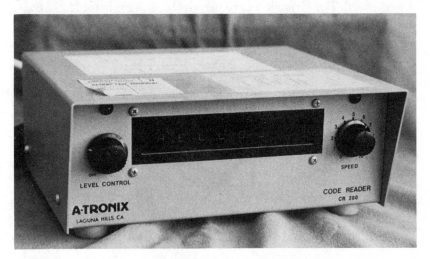

Figure 3–1. A-Tronix keyer.

example, the letter "B" is shown in Figure 3-2 with its code (— . .).
Using this approach, Keith learned all 26 letters, 10 digits, and several
function codes within 3 days.

The second goal was to translate this intellectual association between
codes and letters into motor knowledge. Using the keyer described
earlier, Keith was drilled an hour daily in the codes, beginning with
those that were easiest and progressing to those that required complex
movements. The sequence is shown in Table 3-1.

Third, we worked to increase Keith's tolerance of a faster rate on
the automatic keyer. The goal was to increase his rate without
compromising his accuracy. By the second week on this keyer, Keith
was typing letters in the first two categories on the above chart with
90% accuracy with a keyer rate of 8 words/minute. He continued
practicing the more difficult codes (e.g., the letter C, which is — . — .)
at the slower rate of 5 words/minute.

Operating the Computer with Morse Code

The Adaptive Firmware Card.   By the third week, Keith was able to
sit in his wheelchair long enough to use the Apple Computer for Morse
code practice. This system (see Figs. 3-3 and 3-4) consisted of an Apple
II Plus with the Adaptive Firmware Card produced by Adaptive
Peripherals of Seattle, Washington. Among other functions, this card
allows input of Morse code through the sip-and-puff switch; the
Firmware Card acts as a keyboard emulator in that it translates the
input so that the computer treats that input as if it were directly from
the keyboard. The Firmware Card permits several modes of Morse code,
including standard Morse code, with short "dits" and long "'dahs,"
as well as a code with "dits" and "dahs" of equal length but with tones
of different pitches.

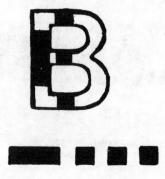

Figure 3-2. Visual mnemonics for Morse code.

We needed to determine which mode would be most appropriate for Keith. After some trials, it became apparent that he could produce the code fastest when the "dits" and "dahs" were equal in length, differing only in pitch of the tone given as feedback. This mode improved Keith's rate and his ability to produce the more difficult codes requiring multiple changes from "sipping" to "puffing."

Increasing the Rate. Keith worked at a slower keyer rate to produce the more difficult codes accurately in isolation. By the end of the fifth week, Keith had mastered the moderately difficult codes such as the letter C (− . − .) but continued having difficulty with the most demanding codes, such as "period" (. − . − . −). Our next goal was

Table 3-1. Sequences of Codes for Training

Codes Requiring One Activation Only:

E	.	T	−
I	. .	M	− −
S	. . .	O	− − −
H	. . . .	BACKSPACE	− − − −
5	. . . . .	0	− − − − −

Codes Requiring Two Activations:

A	. −	N	− .
W	. − −	D	− . .
J	. − − −	B	− . . .
1	. − − − −	6	− . . . .
U	. . −	G	− − .
SPACE	. . − −	Z	− − . .
2	. . − − −	7	− − . . .
V	. . . −	ESCAPE	− − − .
3	. . . − −	8	− − − . .
4	. . . . −	9	− − − − .
REPEAT	. . . . − −	COLON	− − − . . .

Codes Requiring Three Switch Closures:

>	− . − − −	K	− . −
F	. . − .	Q	− − . −
L	. − . .	X	− . . −
P	. − − .	Y	− . − −
R	. − .	COMMA	− − . . − −
?	. . − − . .	HYPHEN	− . . . . −

Codes Requiring More Than Three Closures:

C	− . − .	/	− . . − .
"	. − . − −	)	. . − . −
PERIOD	. − . − . −	SEMICOLON	− . − . − .

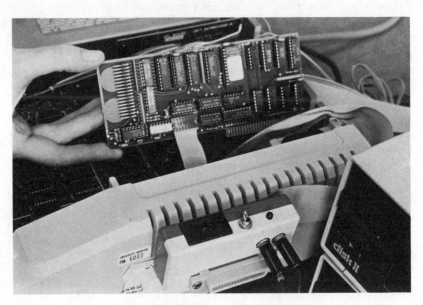

Figure 3-3. Adaptive Firmware Card.

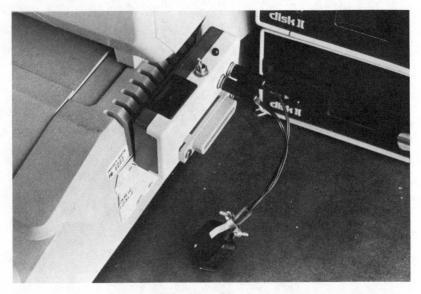

Figure 3-4. Apple II computer with Firmware Card I/O Box.

to increase the rate at which Keith could produce all the codes accurately. In order to accomplish this, we began training letter combinations rather than letters in isolation. Initially, Keith worked on two- and three-letter combinations of the easiest codes. He was to copy words consisting of codes in the first category in Table 3–1, such as "see," "Tom," "meet." Then a second category was added, making words such as "name" and "beam." When he reached the criterion of 85% correct on these tasks we moved on to dictation of these words, sentence completion, and so forth, while gradually increasing the keyer rate. By the end of the fifth week, Keith was using an automatic keyer rate of 14 words/minute for these single words, with 90% accuracy.

Once Keith began to practice at the word level, we measured his "typing" speed. Several factors affected this speed: the automatic keyer rate of the keyboard emulator, Keith's speed of recalling the code, and the number of errors he made while typing. Keith began at a keyer rate of 8 words/minute. That is, if Keith never hesitated in recalling codes and never made any errors, he would have been typing at 8 words/minute. However, these human factors natually affected Keith's typing performance, and we needed to measure Keith's speed in a different manner.

We assessed his overall typing speed on a standard typing test. He was timed on a passage of 100 words, which he was to type as quickly and as accurately as possible. He was to correct all errors as he typed by backspacing and retyping the characters. These corrections greatly slowed his typing speed initially. At the time of this first test, Keith's speed was calculated to be 6.6 words/minute.

At this time, it became apparent that Keith had developed several inappropriate habits that were obstacles to any increase in speed. The first was his reliance on seeing the printed letter on the screen for feedback after each code. Because there was a momentary pause before each letter was displayed, Keith was slowed considerably as he waited for each letter to appear before beginning the next. During this phase, Keith learned to listen to the tone feedback with each "dit" or "dah" that he delivered. He was drilled, facing away from the screen, to recognize correct or incorrect productions using only the auditory and kinesthetic feedback.

Second, Keith had to learn to avoid taking his lips off of the pneumatic tube after each letter. Emphasis was placed on rapid and accurate productions of some of the difficult letter combinations (e.g., "tr," "sch") and the most frequently occurring words in written English. This forced him to think beyond the single letter as he typed. He was given feedback on when he moved his lips from the switch.

Third, Keith had to learn to disassociate his breathing pattern from the activation of the switch. He was drilled on allowing himself to breathe through his nose while he typed a word rather than pausing between words to breathe. At this time, testing showed that Keith's typing speed had increased to 10 words/minute.

Throughout the remaining period of intervention, Keith worked independently to increase his rate and accuracy. By the time of his discharge, Keith's typing speed had increased to 18 words/minute. To type at this speed, he was using the maximum keyer setting on the Firmware Card. Shortly before discharge, the card was modified to permit keyer rates of 30 words/minute and higher, and Keith was inconsistently typing at an actual rate of 20 words/minute. We believe that with additional practice at this keyer speed, Keith could increase his corrected typing rate to 25 words/minute.

SYSTEM SELECTION

Once Keith had become proficient with Morse code, the Division of Vocational Rehabilitation (DVR) expressed an interest in funding equipment. We then made some tentative recommendations regarding appropriate systems for Keith. The team agreed that the speech recognition option, as available in 1982, was not comparable in speed and accuracy to the Morse code approach for several reasons. Speech recognition was limited in the size of vocabulary it could interpret, recognizing approximately 50 words plus the alphabet and punctuation. For report writing, this vocabulary was far too limited, and it would require Keith to spell orally the majority of the words used. This spelling could not be done in the usual "ay, bee, cee, dee" format because the systems could not distinguish between these "words" accurately. Instead, spelling would have to be done using words like "alpha, beta, charlie, delta . . . " For example, the word "bad" would have to be spelled by saying "beta alpha delta." This, coupled with the relatively slow response time of the systems (approximately 1 second for each unit such as "alpha") resulted in an estimated *maximum* speed of 15 words/minute, excluding any time for self-corrections or pauses on the part of the user. Keith had already surpassed that speed with Morse code. For these reasons, it was decided that Keith should use the Morse code approach.

As Keith's job description was clarified, the Apple computer began to appear less adequate to meet his communication needs. The primary disadvantage was thought to be the relatively limited amount of business software available for the Apple. Consultants to the team recommended that we investigate the possibility of a Morse code keyboard emulator for an IBM-PC. Paul Schwejda of Adaptive Peripherals customized such an emulator.

At this point we were ready to submit a tentative list of equipmei. for Keith to DVR. We proposed the following equipment:

1. An IBM-PC with monitor, 64K memory expansion and printer with adapters, cables, and software to support the printer.
2. A hard-disk drive to give Keith independent access to software because he could not change floppy disks.
3. A Prentke Romich sip-and-puff switch.
4. A keyboard emulator, customized by Adaptive Peripherals of Seattle, was to substitute for the Adaptive Firmware Card used during training.
5. A Hayes Smart Modem with serial card and appropriate communications software to allow the PC to receive and transfer information to other computers.
6. Software for word processing and business applications.
7. A Gewa page turner for reading most materials; custom mouthwands and a stand for reading large-sized materials.
8. A Prentke Romich Environmental Control Unit (ECU) for remote control of office equipment.
9. A Prentke Romich Automatic Dialing Telephone (ADT) with an additional sip-and-puff switch.
10. A customized work space to allow independent access via an electric wheelchair to all essential office equipment.
11. Maintenance contracts and insurance for the equipment.

This equipment would meet many of Keith's communication needs. At his office, he would be able to communicate by telephone, operate the Cromemco computer and other computers, write and edit any texts, make and refer to calculations, call up others' reports, make and change diagrams, and compile lists. The equipment would be sufficiently portable to be moved to Keith's home if he were confined to bed for any length of time. However, it would not be portable enough to be moved for short periods of time to allow Keith to take notes at meetings, conferences, or lectures outside his office. A portable cassette recorder would be useful, although it would still not permit Keith to take notes. In addition, this equipment would not allow Keith to make or take phone calls independently when he is out of his office. For the time being, these needs would remain unmet.

At the end of our intervention with Keith, DVR was in the process of reviewing this proposal as well as requests for other personal and transportation equipment. A consultant recommended the following additional equipment:

1. Additional memory to 512K RAM.
2. A 320K floppy disk drive.

3. BSR control modules for remote control of lights and some equipment.
4. Additional business applications software.

This proposal was approved in the spring of 1983. During the summer, the equipment arrived and was fitted into the customized workspace (Fig. 3–5). Keith was back to work on a full-time basis by August 1983, approximately 16 months after his accident.

The team of professionals currently involved with Keith will continue to improve the flexibility and independence of this system. They will be addressing the communication needs not met at the time of this writing. We consider it essential that Keith have a means of working while confined to bed at home because of the frequency of medical complications in quadriplegic patients. In addition, it is important that Keith have a means of taking notes at meetings, lectures, conventions, and a variety of other locations. The team will continue to address such needs.

FOLLOW-UP

At the time this chapter was written, Keith had been back to work for approximately 9 months. He reported that he uses the IBM-PC via Morse code for the majority of his work, in particular because his job description evolved to include a great deal of programming. He is in the process of looking for a second computer, a home computer which will be fully compatible with his IBM at work.

QUESTIONS FOR THE CLINICIAN

Question 1. Why did you select the Morse code system instead of row-column scanning or a direct selection system with a headpointer interface as described in Chapter 2?

Row-column scanning systems are necessarily slower than direct selection systems. They are designed to do most of the "work" by presenting control display options one by one; the user merely waits for the desired option to be offered. This waiting makes the process considerably slower than direct selection. The field of communication augmentation awaits rigorous research comparing the relative efficiency of various interface strategies used by motor impaired individuals.

The optical headpointer, the direct selection system described for Ruby in Chapter 2, was eliminated along with the headwand and

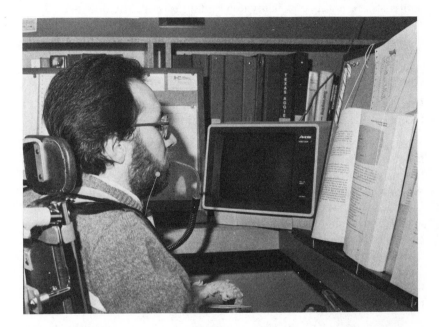

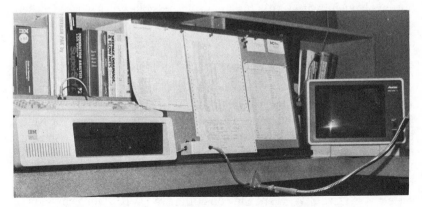

Figure 3–5. Keith's customized workspace.

mouthwand. Keith had lost the function of many neck and shoulder muscles. As a result he fatigues easily in any activities that require fine motor control of the head and neck. Because Keith's job requires him to write throughout his 8-hour workday, these systems were judged to be too fatiguing. Morse code and speech recognition systems, in contrast, are not as physically demanding for an individual like Keith. In addition, Ruby's system requires constant visual contact with the control display. For Keith, Morse code has the advantage that he could review other written materials while producing Morse code, much as other people do as they type.

Question 2.   Do Keith's breathing patterns interfere with his ability to operate the sip-and-puff pneumatic interface?

No. Keith does not control the sip-and-puff switch by maneuvers of the respiratory system but by oral and buccal movements. He changes the air pressure in the oral cavity by subtle lip or tongue movements. As long as he breathes through his nose and not through his mouth, the status of the respiratory system is irrelevant. However, many users approach the sip-and-puff switch as if it were a straw and hold their breath while using it initially. They may require a session or two of training to disassociate the two processes.

Question 3.   How did Keith's employer respond to your proposals regarding such a specialized system for a handicapped employee?

Keith's employer and fellow employees were very receptive to our initial proposal that Keith may be able to return to work. In our first meeting, the team outlined some possible approaches, and Keith's employer described the abilities which Keith would have to have in order to return to full employment with them. Throughout the remainder of our involvement with Keith, his employer and colleagues worked closely with the team to ensure the most appropriate solutions.

ACKNOWLEDGMENTS

It would be impossible to name all the individuals at Harborview Medical Center involved in the development of these systems for Keith. However, the team of individuals who worked most closely with Keith must be mentioned, including Andrea Robertson, OTR; Paul Perkins, Vocational Counselor, and Barbara deLateur, MD, attending physician. In addition, others not associated with the hospital provided additional assistance: Gerald Warren, the consultant to DVR; Paul Schwejda of

Adaptive Peripherals in Seattle; and Howard Christianson of DVR. We must also thank all of Keith's colleagues at Hart Crowser & Associates, who gave so much information and encouragement to allow Keith to return to work there.

REFERENCES

Basic Telecommunications Corporation. *Morse code visual display* (Copyright 1980). 4414 E. Harmony Road, Fort Collins, CO 80525.

Jastak, J.F., and Jastak, S.R. *The Wide Range Achievement Test manual.* Wilmington, DE: Guidance Associates, 1965.

ADDITIONAL READINGS

Donovan, W.H. Spinal cord injury, In W. C. Stolov and M. R. Clowers (Eds.), *Handbook of severe disability.* Washington, DC: US Department of Education, Rehabilitation Services Administration, 1981, pp. 65–82.

McDonald, J.B., Schwejda, P., Marriner, N., Wilson, W., and Ross, A. Advantages of Morse code as a computer input for school-aged children with physical disability. *Computers and the handicapped.* Ottawa: National Research Council of Canada, 1982, pp. 95–106.

Schwejda, P., and Vanderheiden, G.C. Adaptive Firmware Card for the Apple II. *Byte,* 1982, *7,* 276–317.

CHAPTER 4

Loralee

Etiology: Cerebral palsy
Onset: Congenital
Approach: Express III
Focus: This case illustrates the selection decisions and training of a bright child with severe motor control problems. We consider the dual problems of meeting her current communication and educational needs while selecting a system that will not limit her future development.

BACKGROUND

Loralee was referred to our center at the age of 6 years by her pediatrician from the Neuromuscular Disorders Clinic of Children's Orthopedic Hospital, Seattle, and by school district personnel. She was unable to speak owing to severe spastic athetoid cerebral palsy. Our first evaluation of this endearing child was the beginning of our long involvement with Loralee and her many advocates. We have watched Loralee grow and change and we have been involved in the many adjustments that needed to be made in her program to capitalize on her evolving skills.

Intervention for Loralee has never been simple. It has been complicated by a number of factors that required that the program be changed to meet her new communication needs and match her capabilities. Shortly after our first evaluation her needs changed drastically as the school district personnel chose to mainstream Loralee. She was moved into a classroom appropriate for her age because of her strong linguistic skills. Because of her apparent talent, they wanted her to work independently as soon as possible. They were also interested in supplementing her educational experience using a personal computer. In addition to a demanding communication environment, issues of motor control were quite complex, in part because of Loralee's continuing improvement. As you will read in the following sections, Loralee eventually gained some control of her hands, legs, and head. However, none of these interface sites was clearly superior to the others. Although the promise of multiple switch control was present, the child's level of "motor thinking" was not adequate for multiple switch control. Such control needed to be developed step by step. Because of Loralee's apparent potential, she received extensive training, especially in the area of motor control. Eventually her level of cooperation began to ebb. Both her physical therapist and speech-language pathologist reported a lack of compliance with treatment activities. Finally, Loralee's intervention was complex because it involved much more technical equipment than school personnel had used previously. These factors made intervention in Loralee's case challenging for all involved. It meant that recommendations regarding equipment and intervention were never either final or complete.

Early Communication Approaches

Loralee's communication systems evolved as she grew, beginning with a simple picture board, which was introduced when she was 2 years old. Photographs were used as the initial symbol set. Gradually, the photos were replaced with line drawings and then with words. By the time she was 5 years old, Loralee was proficient at responding with the 200-word communication board. This approach required that she first indicate the general area of the board through eye gaze or arm movement. Then her partner would "scan" through the items in that area, asking whether each item was the one she intended. Loralee would signal her choice with a slight head nod.

School History

Prior to our evaluation of Loralee, the local school district had completed an extensive assessment. She scored within normal limits on the Test of Auditory Comprehension of Language (Carrow, 1973), the Peabody Picture Vocabulary Test (Dunn, 1965), and several subtests of the Illinois Test of Psycholinguistic Abilities (McCarthy and Kirk, 1961). Other tests showed that her reading and spelling skills were at or above age level. She showed deficits only in mathematics, as measured by the Peabody Individual Achievement Test (Dunn and Markwardt, 1970). Her expressive language was not assessed.

Loralee was mainstreamed into a regular first grade classroom with an aide and a resource room available to her. According to all reports, she was functioning at or above grade level in all academic areas. She attended class in a Mulholland wheelchair, fitted with special head and trunk supports. The word board and a buzzer to call attention were mounted on her laptray. The buzzer was also used to respond to questions involving mathematics.

In speech treatment, Loralee used the word board to answer questions and to formulate sentences on request. According to all reports, she did not use the board in spontaneous communication in any other environment. The board served primarily as an academic tool. Her day-to-day communication was managed through eye gaze, "twenty questions," the buzzer to call attention, and head nodding. Loralee had been trained in single switch use with a leaf switch to activate a mechanical toy dog and the buzzer already mentioned. After she had become proficient with this switch, training began on a Zygo 16 row-column scanner (Fig. 4–1) in the Step Scan mode. Each time the switch was depressed the scanning light moved one location. According to school reports, Loralee was not able to use a headwand or a headlight pointer; nor was she able to use a rocking lever switch placed at her foot, knee, or hand or under her chin.

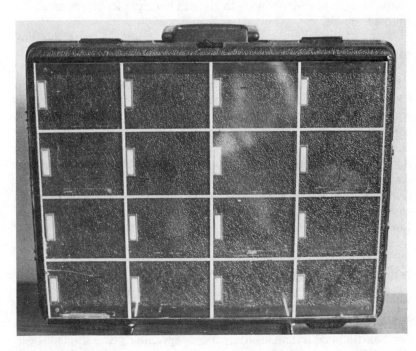

Figure 4–1. The Zygo 16 row-column scanner (manufactured by Zygo Industries, Inc., Portland, OR).

INITIAL EVALUATION

The evaluation at our center was arranged by her pediatrician to answer a variety of questions. The caregivers were particularly interested in the best control interface for Loralee, the most appropriate scanning system, and some recommendations in training on such devices and their integration into the classroom.

Assessment

Loralee was initially seen at our center in May 1982 at age 6 years. Her motor control was evaluated in the criterion-based manner described in Chapter 1. Her hand control was inadequate for direct selection. Evaluation of head control showed that she had greater head control for horizontal movements than for vertical movements. Her poor control of vertical movements precluded the use of a headlight pointer. However, her control of horizontal movements appeared sufficient for control of bilateral pressure switches. Movements of her head to the right were more reliable than movements to the left, which were associated with occasional asymmetric tonic neck reflex (ATNR). She consistently was able to elevate the toes of her right foot by dorsiflexing the right ankle.

Recommendations

It was obvious that Loralee was not yet ready to control a communication system with the bilateral head switches. Therefore, it was recommended that she receive intensive motor training in switch control. The "Motor Training Games" developed for the Apple Computer by Judy McDonald and Paul Schwejda were recommended for this training. In addition, it was suggested that Loralee receive training in reading, spelling, and other language arts skills through selected computer games. The school district was encouraged to continue stressing the spelling, reading, and syntactical aspects of Loralee's language arts program, as they had in the past.

SECOND EVALUATION

In July 1983 Loralee, now 7 years old, returned to our center for a follow-up evaluation in conjunction with her annual appointment with her Seattle pediatrician. During the intervening year, she had been fitted with a new wheelchair with trunk supports and a halo for vertical head support (Fig. 4-2).

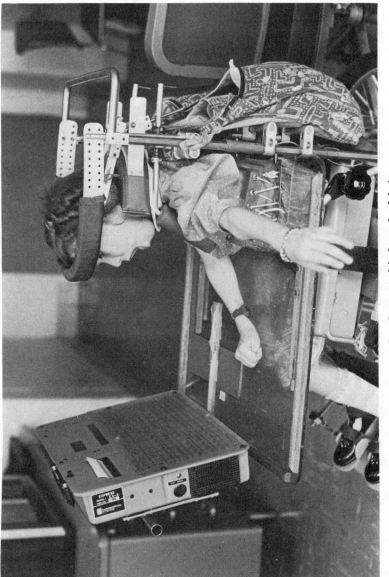

Figure 4 – 2. Loralee seated in her wheelchair.

Physical therapy and language instruction in the school had progressed well after the computer was introduced. Loralee's cooperation in her motor control program increased dramatically when the Motor Training games were utilized. Training was directed specifically toward improving motor control with bilateral head switches manufactured by Zygo Industries, Inc.

In our evaluation, Loralee demonstrated that she had improved markedly in her control of the head switches. She demonstrated the ability to activate either switch on command without error, to avoid hitting either switch when instructed to wait, and to activate the two switches in rapid succession. She showed some overflow movements, but these were reduced when the switches were moved closer to her head on both sides. Moving the switches closer also reduced the excursion required to activate them, thereby allowed her to watch more easily a control display while activating the switches.

Loralee continued to use the word board as her primary means of communication. She was now able to indicate the column of words with her right hand, a more efficient approach for her than eye-gaze. The listener then scanned the words in the column verbally and Loralee indicated.

During the previous year, an Express III had become available to Loralee, and the decision was made to give her a trial with it (see Chapter 2 for a description of the Express III system). An attempt was made to have Loralee operate the Express system in a row-column, interrupted scanning mode. In this mode the scanning light travels sequentially from row to row. The user activates a switch to select the preferred row and the horizontal column scan begins. The switch is reactivated to collect the preferred location. This mode caused a marked increase in Loralee's athetoid movements. As the scanning light approached a location of choice, the movements increased so that she was unable to accurately activate a switch. During a trial in the "directed" scan mode, in which the scanning light moves only when the switch was depressed, Loralee's athetoid movements were less excessive, and she was able to release the switch to indicate her choices. Because she could activate only two switches, it was recommended that she control the Express via directed scanning with timed acceptance. This means that she would move the cursor vertically or horizontally with the two switches stopping on the desired location. That location would be accepted after the cursor had remained there for the specified length of time. Initially the timed acceptance was slow, permitting Loralee to hesitate while moving the cursor to the desired location. It was assumed that later, as she became more proficient with the switches, the acceptance rate would be increased. When Loralee was able to control a third switch, she would no longer need to use timed acceptance. The third switch could serve to "accept" the location of the cursor. This would undoubtably increase Loralee's communication rate. It was also recommended that the Express III be programmed to make the individual units on the control display larger in size than the standard single square. This would increase Loralee's accuracy initially, in that target areas would be made up of four squares rather than a single square. As her motor control and motor planning improved, the targets could be made smaller. When Loralee was able to control the hand switch to signal acceptance, it was possible to abandon the timed acceptance that she had been using. In addition, she learned to control foot switch (Fig. 4–3) that could be used to move

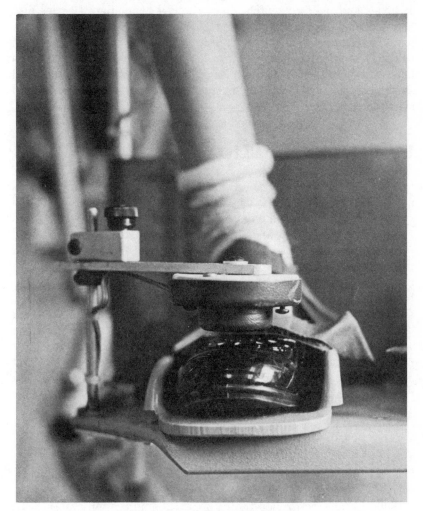

Figure 4–3. Loralee's footswitch.

the cursor in the vertical dimension. The head switches could be used for control in the horizontal directions, allowing her to move the cursor both left and right. These dual horizontal directions increased efficiency because she no longer had to move the light "around the back of the unit" to the desired location.

THIRD EVALUATION

Loralee returned for a reevaluation 3 months later. During the intervening months the school had trained her to control the two head switches and the foot switch. Since the last evaluation, Loralee also had developed the ability to control a switch with her right hand. A hand switch was mounted in her lap tray. A training program was begun to teach Loralee four switch control of the Express system. The two head switches controlled left and right horizontal movement; the hand switch controlled vertical movement; and the foot switch was used to signal acceptance.

FOURTH EVALUATION

Although Loralee was able to control each of the four switches independently, she had difficulty learning to control the communication system using them in combination. Her control of the left head switch was much more accurate and efficient than her control of the right head switch. During attempts at system operation, she frequently activated the right head switch inadvertently. She also demonstrated difficulty remembering to use the foot switch as an "acceptance" switch. The four switch appeared too complex, and a simplified motor access strategy was implemented. The right head switch was removed and the system was programmed to scan to the left on the horizontal plane when the left head switch was depressed (Fig. 4–4). Loralee no longer had a switch that would move the scanning light in the left-to-right direction. Loralee directed the light "around the back" of the Express to access locations on the right-hand side of the control display. The hand switch was used to move the light in a vertical direction. She could only move the light from top to bottom, going "around the back" of the device to access choices on the top of the control display. The acceptance of selections was made with an additional hand switch located to the right of the switch used for vertical movement of the scanning light (Fig. 4–5).

While Loralee controlled the Express Communication system with three switches, her physical therapy program continued to stress her

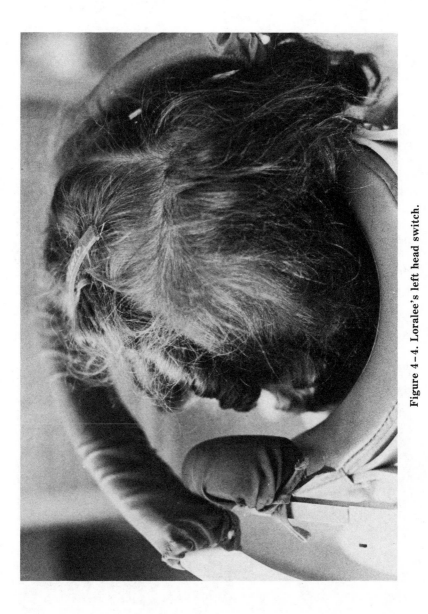

Figure 4-4. Loralee's left head switch.

use of the other switches as well. It is hoped that as she becomes more familiar with switch control she will have a variety of motor control choices for communication system, computer, page turner, and wheelchair control.

CURRENT STATUS

At the time this chapter was written, Loralee had operated the Express Communication system in her classroom at school for approximately 8 weeks. She uses the system primarily as a "pencil" in that she practices spelling words and completes mathematics and writing assignments. She uses two overlays with her communication system. One is a general writing overlay which contains letters and commonly occurring words. The second is a mathematics overlay with numbers, mathematical symbols, and requests for assistance. Although Loralee still uses an educational aide, her teacher is very positive about the use of the communication augmentation system in the classroom.

Now that Loralee has begun to use the system in the classroom, personnel from the school district and our center are beginning to focus on Loralee's use of the interactive capabilities of the system. For now,

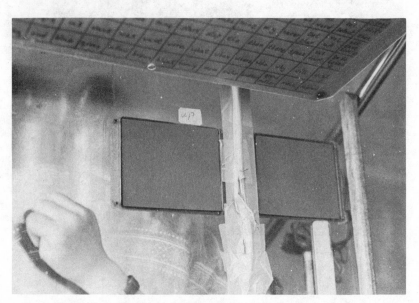

Figure 4-5. Two hand switches mounted in Loralee's laptray.

this will be accomplished through two activities. First, we are developing an overlay that contains the alphabet and many conversational control phases. Currently, Loralee, her family, school district staff, and center staff are compiling a master list of phrases, which will gradually be entered into the Express III and displayed on a "conversational" overlay. Second, we are developing overlays that will assist Loralee to interact as she plays games with family and friends. To begin with, we are developing an overlay that will assist her to play UNO, her favorite card game. In addition, we are developing an overlay to play "dolls" with the help of her mother and sister. Our goal is to have the academic, conversational, UNO, and "doll" overlays ready for the summer vacation. If Loralee can use her communication system productively over the summer, she may be ready to begin to use the system as a computer keyboard emulator during the fall. Undoubtedly, her instruction in using the system for effective conversational interaction will continue for years as she matures and her communication needs change.

QUESTIONS FOR THE CLINICIAN

Question 1. Why did you decide on a scanning system rather than waiting until Loralee's spelling and motor control would allow a trial with a Morse code–based system?

The school personnel were becoming increasingly concerned that Loralee have a communication system to support her academic program. If we had waited for Loralee to develop the motor control to access a Morse code–based system, she might have fallen behind her classmates in the very skills required for this system.

The Express III was selected over other scannning systems for several reasons. First, the numerous control and process options make it flexible, and this is ideal for someone whose motor control is continuing to develop. As Loralee's motor control changed, the system could be controlled with one, two, three, four, or five switches. The function of each switch could be defined and the device could be set up for timed acceptance or manual acceptance. In Loralee's case we made use of this flexibility. As we served her, Loralee's motor capability changed. The Express system accommodated the changes. In retrospect, we would not ask the usual young communication augmentation system user to make the number of changes which Loralee experienced during a short period of time. The availability of motor control alternatives as well as the pressure from parents and school district personnel to provide the potentially most rapid system possible led to a period of time when several different switch control approaches are attempted. In addition, this system allowed for the potential use of a optical headpointer for direct selection if her head control improved. The second reason for this system choice was that the school personnel were very concerned that Loralee be able to access conventional computer software through her communication system. The Express purchased for Loralee contains a keyboard emulator for the Apple II computer. After she has developed the motor control and motor learning required for efficient use of the Express III as a communication system, we will begin her training in its use as a keyboard for the Apple II.

Question 2.   How did the school district personnel deal with the use of such a complex communication system in an academic training program?

School personnel were wonderfully supportive of Loralee and her need for a communication system. At times their eagerness to serve Loralee resulted in expectations which our center, and even Loralee, were unable to meet in a timely manner. When the Express III arrived, there was a push to implement the system for communication immediately in all environments. It was necessary to reduce these expectations, so that Loralee would have sufficient time to become proficient in using the system. She needed to learn the motor control features of the system, learn system operations, and then learn to do elementary message preparation before the system could be expected to meet a broad variety of communication needs. A mistake on the part of our center staff was that we did not provide better training for the school personnel in the use of the Express III soon after it was delivered. The school staff experienced intense frustration in the early days with the system. Coupled with their high expectations, the lack of system information could have been a serious impediment to our intervention with Loralee. However, a few meetings with the entire team allowed us to deal systematically with most of these problems shortly after they arose.

Question 3.   What is "motor thinking" and why is it important?

Judy McDonald introduced the concept of "motor thinking" in relation to communication augmentation. Motor thinking is the ability to predict the consequences of motor activity such that the intended outcome is achieved. For example, motor thinking is an important part of learning to drive a car. Most "new" drivers have the motor control to turn the steering wheel but they must learn the motor thinking involved in parallel parking. In communication augmentation the user must learn to predict the effect of switch closure, joystick movement, and head position if the system is to be controlled accurately and efficiently. Most communication augmentation system users with congenital impairment have had limited motor experience because of their severe motor disability.

Often physical therapy, occupational therapy, and recreational time must be used to provide them with experience in motor thinking to prepare them for subsequent system use. Practice is critical in developing motor thinking. This point can be illustrated by considering the difference between the "conceptual" and "motor learning" require to operate an interface. Conceptually the user needs to understand that, for example, activating the right switch moves the light to the right, the left switch moves the light to the left and the foot switch moves the light up. Conceptual learning can take place in one trial. The motor learning required to perform this task, on the other hand, may require thousands of repetitions before the motor pattern is established.

Question 4. In Chapter 1 you present a figure in which you outline the selection decision that come from the evaluation process. How does the selection of a system for a child with changing needs and capability fit into this model?

The process described in Figure 1–1 can be thought of as a snapshot capturing the selection decisions at one point in time for an individual with stable communication needs and capabilities. Of course, the decision-making process becomes much more complex when making selection decisions for a child like Loralee, for whom we expect that both communication needs and capabilities will change in many important ways over a period of years. In selecting an augmentation approach for a child, we ask two general questions. The first is, "How can today's communication be maximized?" The second question is, "How will future communication needs most effectively be met?"

For today, we use the selection decision process as is outlined in Figure 1–1. The communication needs are identified and capabilities assessed, and then a series of approaches are developed that best meet the current needs of the child. Often multiple approaches are identified. Selection decisions made for a child with developing needs and capabilities are often more complex than those for an individual with stable needs and capabilities. When selecting an approach for a child, you must also plan for the future by asking questions like, "Are the approaches selected for today part of a sequence that will lead to more effective future approaches?" For Loralee, today's system was chosen so that it would allow her to make maximum use of her developing motor control skills by moving to ever larger numbers of switch options. It was also selected so that it would not restrict the development of her language and academic abilities. For today, the system could be programmed as a word or phrase retrieval system; for tomorrow, it could be used as a typing system whereby she could create unique messages in a letter-by-letter fashion. For today, academic work could focus on the development of spelling and language formulation skills. In the future, Loralee could use the system for computer access to a wide range of academic software. With children, the selection of communication augmentation systems involves not only the periodic reassessment of changing communication needs and capabilities but also prediction of future peformance.

ACKNOWLEDGMENTS

Loralee's intervention was an interdisciplinary, multiple agency effort. Thanks must go to the staffs of The Neuromuscular Disorder Clinic of Children's Orthopedic Hospital, Seattle, and the Yakima, Washington, School District. Of special note, Linda Crossland was the coordinator of the School District's effort. Wendell Matas of Rehab Equipment, Seattle, resolved numerous technical issues.

REFERENCES

Carrow, E. *Test of auditory comprehension of language.* Austin, TX: Learning Concepts, 1973.

Dunn, L. M. *Expanded manual for the Peabody Picture Vocabulary Test.* Circle Pines, MN: American Guidance Service, 1965.

Dunn, L. M., and Markwardt, W. H. *Peabody Individual Achievement Test.* Circle Pines, MN: American Guidance Service, 1970.

McCarthy, J. J., and Kirk, S. A. *Illinois Test of Psycholinguistic Abilities.* Urbana, IL: University of Illinois Institute for Research on Exceptional Children, 1961.

ADDITIONAL READINGS

Fountain Valley School District. *Nonoral communication: A training guide to the child without speech.* Fountain Valley, CA, 1980.

McDonald, E.T., and Schultz, A.R. Communication boards for cerebral-palsied children. *Journal of Speech and Hearing Disorders*, 1973, *38*, 73–88.

CHAPTER 5

Debbie

Etiology: Cerebral palsy
Onset: Congenital
Approach: Epson HX-20 and Star Gemini-X10 Printer
Focus: This chapter focuses on a computer-based writing system for a college student with cerebral palsy. The Epson HX-20 computer was selected as the core unit of the system. Implementation of computer systems in academic settings is discussed.

BACKGROUND

Debbie, a 26 year old woman with moderately severe athetoid cerebral palsy, was referred to our center by the staff of her junior college. They were concerned about a number of educational and communication needs related to the mainstreaming of severely physically handicapped individuals into college settings. Debbie was able to manage most interpersonal communication through speech. On the Assessment of Intelligibility of Dysarthric Speech (Yorkston and Beukelman, 1981), she achieved a sentence intelligibility score of 86% at a speaking rate of 90 words per minute. She reported that occasionally, strangers did not understand her, but that she usually resolved breakdowns verbally. Debbie had learned to write using an electric typewriter. During her early elementary years, she had used a keyguard, but in junior high school she had begun to type without it. Her typing rate was 12 words/minute. Debbie could not walk and used a manual wheelchair, which she propelled with her feet. She required no special lateral or anterior trunk supports in the chair.

EVALUATION

Capability Assessment

Motor Control. Debbie demonstrated access to an electric typewriter by depressing the keys with the index finger of her right hand. Although she also was able to depress keys with the middle and little fingers of her right hand, her typing rate was reduced when she attempted multiple finger typing over that obtained with single finger typing. She had difficulty in protruding the finger of choice and in extending or flexing the remaining fingers to avoid inadverent key strokes. With this difficulty, multiple finger typing did not offer an increase in typing efficiency. Although unable to type accurately with her left hand, she could depress the shift key with her left thumb as she depressed letter and number keys with her right hand. Because Debbie was able to control a direct selection interface with acceptable rate and accuracy, we did not evaluate her potential for joystick or single switch control.

Vision.   Debbie's optometrist reported that her visual acuity was corrected with glasses and that she had no other visual problems.

Language and Cognition.   Debbie had successfully completed high school. Information from a number of language and academic achievement tests were available to us. On the Peabody Picture Vocabulary test (Dunn, 1965), she achieved a receptive vocabulary age at the ceiling of the test (18.5 years). On the Gates-MacGinitie Reading Test (Gates and MacGinitie, 1965, 1969), she scored at the 8.8 grade equivalent level. On the Wide Range Achievement Test (Jastak and Jastak, 1965), she received a spontaneous spelling grade equivalent score of 6.0.

Communication Needs

As was mentioned previously, Debbie's speech was adequate to meet most interpersonal communication needs. Her primary unmet needs involved writing activities related to her participation in a local junior college. She was interested in learning computer programming in addition to completing the work associated with other academic classes. A specific list of her communication needs are presented in Table 5–1. In summary, Debbie needed a flexible writing system, which would be portable, so that she could take notes in several different classrooms during the day and prepare assignments during breaks. At the same time the system was needed for programming practice and computer access.

RECOMMENDATIONS

The System

The Computer.   We selected the Epson HX-20 portable computer (Fig. 5–1) as the core element of our writing system for Debbie. This system,

Table 5–1. Mandatory Communication Augmentation Needs For Debbie

Message Types:
> Prepare unique messages
> Prepare formal paper in 8½ by 11 inch format
> Take notes in class (any format)
> Write memos (any format)
> Write letters

Environments:
> Various college classrooms
> College library
> On the bus

Communication Partners:
> College faculty
> College students
> Friends and family

Special Needs:
> Access to college computers
> The system should allow Debbie to practice programming at college and at home

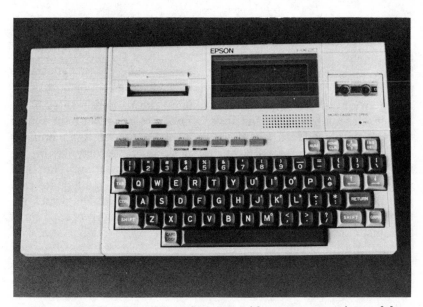

Figure 5–1. The Epson HX-20 Computer with memory expansion module.

with its memory expansion module, is highly portable, weighing 3 pounds and measuring 12.5 by 8.5 by 2 inches. The internal batteries power the system for up to 70 hours of use per recharge. The basic system contains a screen (four lines of 24 characters each), a strip printer (20 characters per line), and a microcassette tape drive for storage. The memory expansion module increases the memory of the system from 16 to 32 K. In addition, the Epson HX-20 comes equipped with the Skiwriter chip, which provides the unit with excellent word processing software.

Word Processing.   Our plan included Debbie's use of the Skiwriter program to support her note taking in class and her paper and letter writing activities. With the microcassette storage system, Debbie could work on several different projects without requiring the help of someone else to store her work for her. The cassette storage system permits the user to store three different writing projects on a single side of a microcassette.

Printing.   By itself, the Epson computer could not meet several of Debbie's communication needs. For example, she would be unable to print her written assignments in 8 1/2 by 11 inch format. We purchased a Star Gemini-10X printer for her along with the cable to connect the computer and the printer. This printer is left at Debbie's home. She does all of her formal report and letter printing there.

Mounting.   The mounting of Debbie's writing system is shown in Figure 5–2. This mounting is designed to serve several purposes. First, the computer is secured, so it will not fall from Debbie's wheelchair laptray as she moves from place to place. Second, the system is protected by the case that surrounds it. Third, an extension for the off/on switch of the computer is built into the mounting (Fig. 5–3). Debbie does not have the hand and finger control to activate the switch that is a standard feature of the Epson HX-20. Fourth, the mounting can be adjusted to raise and lower the position of the computer on the lapboard and to tilt the keyboard for optimal position. The final adaptation of Debbie's system was the provision of an adequate rain guard. As Debbie moves about the campus and as she waits for transportation, she frequently gets caught in rain. An occupational therapist at our center developed a vinyl rain cover, which has worked successfully for several months.

Training

Debbie's instruction with the system was provided at our center during once-weekly sessions. She was accompanied by her father, who

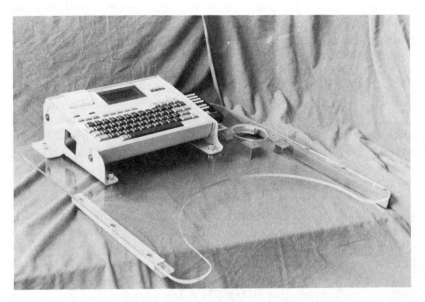

Figure 5-2. The mounting system for the Epson HX-20.

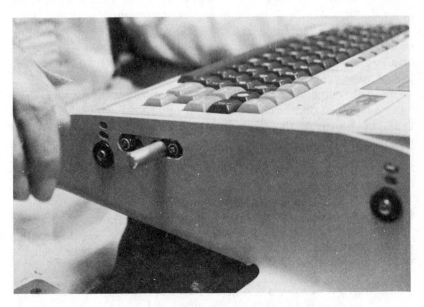

Figure 5-3. The off/on switch modification.

was very interested in her system. Together, Debbie and her father studied the tutorial booklets provided with the Epson HX-20 computer and the Skiwriter software. After the first several familiarization sessions, we spent most of our time working with Debbie to plan her management of various writing assignments and note-taking activities, so that she would have storage room on the microcassette and in the memory of the computer for a day of writing and note taking.

One feature of the Epson HX-20 computer enhances its capability as a writing system. The "CMOS" memory of the system permits the storage of the program and data even when the computer is switched off. Of course, the microcassette can be used to store three different writing projects, each about 15 pages in length. Since the Skiwriter program is stored on a chip, it does not occupy storage space on the microcassette.

After one month of use, Debbie was able to type at a rate of 12 words/minute. She demonstrated understanding of the basic functions of system control, such as the built-in printer, microcassette storage system, off/on, and recharge. She used the Skiwriter word processing program very effectively for note taking and paper writing. At the time this chapter was written, she was learning about peripheral printer control and formatting with the Skiwriter program.

Computer Access.   As was apparent from Debbie's needs list, she required access to computers on which she could learn and practice programming. At this stage she does some programming on the Epson HX-20, however, she finds that the small screen makes programming somewhat difficult. She is unable to view the lines of code as she could on a larger screen. As her programming skills improve, this limitation will become even more confining.

One of the computers in the computer laboratory in her junior college has been placed on a special table that allows her wheelchair access to the keyboard. At this time, she requires assistance to remove her laptray and to insert her program disks into the disk drive of the college computer. If she were working on her own system, a hard disk would reduce this problem.

QUESTIONS FOR THE CLINICIAN

Question 1.   Why did you select the Epson HX-20 rather than the Radio Shack TRS-80, Model 100?

The primary reason we selected the Epson HX-20 computer was the reliable microcassette system for storing text and programs. In addition, the built-in printer allows Debbie to prepare memos and short answer assignments in written form. The Model 100 has neither a build-in storage system nor a printer. One advantage of the model 100 is the larger built-in screen size compared with the Epson HX-20.

Question 2. Why did you select a computer system rather than one of the portable lightweight battery-powered typewriters that are now available commercially?

In many applications in which a writing system is required, a portable typewriter would be adequate. We did not make this selection for Debbie because of her heavy writing requirements as well as her interest in computer programming. As time goes by and Debbie's writing requirements change, we hope to continue to individualize her software programs and provide her with a variety of capabilities, including software, which would function as a daily, weekly, and yearly calendar and address and phone book. With younger students who require a portable writing system, but as of yet do not have extensive writing requirements, we frequently recommend the Sharp El-7100 or the Expanded Keyboard Sharp (see Chapter 8).

Question 3. Is there a way to equip the Epson computer so that regular disk drives and a large monitor can be used?

Obviously, if standard disk drives and a large monitor could be used with the Epson HX-20, both word processing and programming could be managed more effectively. As we were completing the manuscript for this book, both of these options were becoming available. Although our local Epson representative assures us that these options are workable, we have had no experience with them.

Question 4. Are there research and development efforts being undertaken that will enhance the Epson HX-20 computer as a writing and computer control aid?

Three current efforts should be mentioned. Adaptive Peripherals of Seattle is developing a keyboard emulator or keyboard link between the Epson HX-20 and Apple computers containing an Adaptive Peripherals Firmware Card (see the Glossary for a discussion of the Firmware Card). The keyboard link will allow an Epson user to access an Apple computer and operate unmodified software programs on it. This application was not necessary for Debbie, because she was able to access an unmodified personal computer keyboard. However, for the individual requiring a specialized keyboard control or Morse code–type control of the Epson HX-20 computer, the keyboard link to the Apple computer will permit access to school or business computers without altering the mounting or keyboard setup used by nonimpaired students or staff.

Second, Adaptive Peripherals has developed a module to translate Morse code into English and act as a keyboard emulator for the Epson HX-20. The module is positioned in the memory expansion module of the Epson HX-20. The electrical connectors from the interface switches are inserted into the side of the memory module (Fig. 5–4).

Words+, Inc., of Sunnyvale, California has developed single and double switch Morse code translation capability for the Epson HX-20 Computer. At the time this chapter was written, the Words+ approach utilized the working memory of the Epson rather than a keyboard emulation approach to accomplish Morse code translation.

Third, the Trace Center at the University of Wisconsin, Madison, is engaged in an active research program to utilize the Epson HX-20 as a portable electronic writing, conversation, and computer access aid. Specifically, the Trace proposal includes the development of the following functions: calculator, dictionary, environmental control, keyboard emulator, worksheet, and notebook. A message preparation

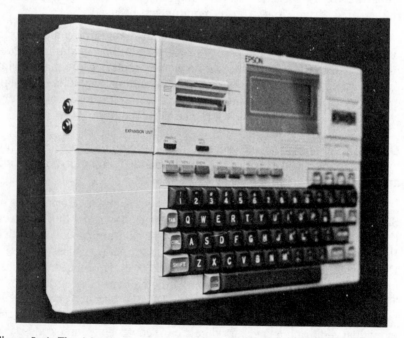

Figure 5–4. The Adaptive Peripherals modification to the memory expansion of module of the Epson HX-20.

rate enhancement program called "speedkey" will also be included. The "speedkey" function in its most advanced form automatically replaces an abbreviation with the associated expansion. For example, the word "definition" could be represented by the character string "dfn." The three characters used to represent the word "definition" are related to the word by extracting key consonants.

Question 5. Do you expect that computer accessibility for individuals with severe physical disabilities will increase their educational and vocational potential?

It is very easy to answer with an unqualified "yes." However, our early experience causes us to be somewhat more reserved. Several concerns are becoming apparent as students equipped with sophisticated communication equipment or computers, or both, enter school at a variety of levels. First, many physically disabled indivduals have fairly limited academic backgrounds for many reasons, including lack of efficient communication approaches, amount of time needed in focusing on nonacademic concerns, such as physical control, poor attendence for health reasons, and reduced academic expectations. This lack of academic preparation may be reflected in reduced spontaneous spelling ability, lack of experience with written expression, reduced mathematical abilities, and so forth. The purchase of a computer or sophisticated communication system does not eliminate the academic weaknesses.

Second, even with sophisticated equipment, many physically disabled individuals find it difficult to compete in an academic program with nonimpaired students. Several of the school districts that are attempting to serve junior and senior high school students who have severe physical disabilities are struggling with the reduced efficiency of these students. In many cases, the school district hoped that the communication or computer system would eliminate the need for a human aide in the educational process. In most instances, this has not been the case. While the communication system has allowed greater independence on the part of the disabled student, the pace of a normal junior or senior high school requires that the students be provided with whatever tools are necessary if they are expected to compete academically. In addition, the school, student, and family need to coordinate homework, computer assisted instruction, and summer school to maximize the educational preparation of the physically disabled student. When there was no expectation that a student would compete educationally or vocationally, some of the issues mentioned earlier were less urgent. In short, the availability to sophisticated systems has at the same time reduced dependency but increased expectation.

Third, our experience with communication augmentation system users in the workplace is very limited. Keith, whose care was discussed in Chapter 3, appears to have made a successful return to his job. However, he had a established work history prior to his injury and had an employer who was very supportive of his efforts. Keith is not alone; others are making the transition into vocations in ever-increasing numbers. This trend is wonderful, yet it takes careful planning and preparation.

ACKNOWLEDGMENTS

We wish to thank Marvin Soderquist for development of the mounting system.

REFERENCES

Dunn, L. M. *Expanded manual for the Peabody Picture Vocabulary Test.* Circle Pines, MN: Americian Guidance Service, 1965.

Gates, A. I., and MacGinitie, W. H. *Gates-MacGinitie Reading Test.* New York: Teacher's College Press, Columbia University, 1965, 1969.

Jastak, J. F., and Jastak, S. R. *Wide Range Achievement Test.* Wilmington, DE: Guidance Associates, 1965.

Yorkston, K. M., and Beukelman, D. R. *Assessment of intelligibility of dysarthric speech.* Tigard, OR: C. C. Publications, 1981.

ADDITIONAL READINGS

Traynor, C. D., and Beukelman, D.R. Nonvocal communication augmentation using microcomputers. *Exceptual Education Quarterly*, 1984, *4*, 90–103.

Vanderheiden, G. C. Computers can play a dual role for disabled individuals. *Byte*, 1982, *7*, 136–165.

Vanderheiden, G. C. Technology needs of indivudals with communication impairments. *Seminars in Speech and Language*, 1984, *5*, 59–67.

CHAPTER 6

Steve

Etiology: Spinal cord injury, cervical level 1-2 (C1-2)
Onset: 32 years of age
Approach: Eye-gaze System
Electrolarynx
Tracheostomy cuff deflation
Voice amplifier
Computer-based writing system
Focus: This chapter illustrates the case of a spinal cord–injured, respirator-dependent adult. We describe the transition through a series of communication augmentation approaches until Steve was able to speak. A computer-based writing system controlled via a sip-and-puff interface is also described.

BACKGROUND

Steve is a 32 year old man who suffered a gunshot wound to his neck. He was not breathing when the paramedics found him and was sustained by respiratory bagging enroute to the hospital. The gunshot wound to his right neck damaged his right external carotid artery and severed his spinal cord at the level of the first cervical vertebra. As a consequence of his spinal cord injury, Steve had no motor control below his chin; he had no control over his neck muscles and was unable to move his shoulders, arms, or legs. Because his diaphragm was paralyzed bilaterally, a tracheotomy was performed and Steve was supported with a respirator. He was unable to produce a voice because of the cuffed tracheostomy. Neuromotor control of the oral speech musculature was intact, but the lymphatic flow from the area was disrupted and his tongue swelled to the extent that precise oral speech movements were not possible.

Early Communication Approaches. Steve initially communicated via an eye blink "yes/no" signal system, blinking once to indicate "no" and raising his eyebrows slightly to indicate "yes." This was supplemented a short time later with an eye-gaze system by the speech–language pathologist at the hospital where Steve received his acute medical care. An eye-gaze system is illustrated in Figure 6–1. It consists of a clear plastic sheet with a center cut-out. The size of the system is approximately 30 by 32 inches. The system can be positioned over a bed on a stand or placed on a hospital table over the bed. Letters, words, or phrases can be mounted at nine locations by means of clips. In order to use the system, communication partners stood in a position so that they could look through the board and watch Steve's eye movements. He directed his gaze to the location of the desired letter or message. When there were multiple entries at each locations, the partner scanned the possiblities and Steve selected the appropriate one by indicating "yes." Steve's initial system contained the alphabet, medical needs, such as the need for suctioning, and personal messages, such as names of family members. The speech-language pathologist's report indicated that Steve was able to use the eye-gaze system successfully within the limits of his tolerance of fatigue. He did not appear to have difficulty reading the words and phrases used on the board, nor did he have difficulty spelling out short messages.

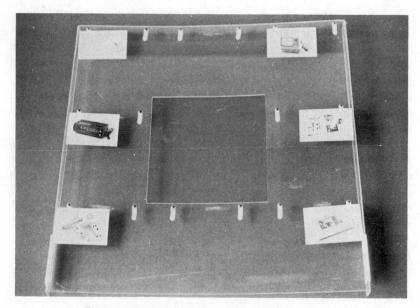

Figure 6–1. An eye-gaze communication system.

INITIAL EVALUATION

Status on Admission to Rehabilitation. Steve's acute medical care was provided in a hospital in another state. He was transferred to our setting for rehabilitation and exploration of the potential for implantation of a phrenic nerve pacer. He was admitted to our rehabilitation unit approximately 3 months after the injuury. At that time he had just recovered from an episode of pneumonia. He remained respirator-dependent with the tracheotomy cuff inflated at all times. Figure 6–2 (left) provides a schematic representation of the inflated cuff. A review of this figure illustrates that all of the ventilatory air is directed into the lungs, and none is allowed to pass through the vocal folds for voice production. The cuff inflation is necessary for those patients who do not have respiratory stability. The closed system provided by the inflated cuff allows respiratory specialists to monitor respiratory pressure and flow accurately to ensure adequate ventilatory exchange. The inflated cuff also minimizes the risk of aspiration of oral secretions or food for patients with swallowing difficulty.

Communication Needs Assessment

Initially the assessment of Steve's communication needs was carried out in two phases. The first phase involved asking the question, "What

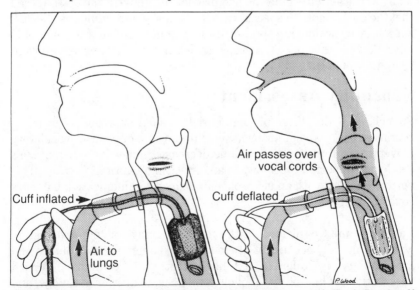

Air passes over vocal cords

Cuff inflated

Cuff deflated

Air to lungs

Figure 6–2. A schematic representation of a tracheostomy cuff. The inflated cuff (left) prevents ventilatory air from passing through the vocal folds. The deflated cuff (right) allows the patient to produce a voice as the ventilatory air is passed through the vocal folds.

are the mandatory communication functions which are required for today?" The second phase involved questions about the future: "What tasks will Steve need for maximal functioning at the time of discharge?"

Current Needs. For the present, Steve needed an accurate, rapid, nonfatiguing means of communicating with the hospital staff. He needed to communicate quickly a small number of relatively predictable messages. He also needed to answer short questions and occasionally produce a long unique message. The eye-gaze system, although it was successful in that Steve could communicate his messages, proved frustrating for both Steve and his communication partners. It was an extremely slow approach which required a good deal of patience. Steve needed to tolerate poor retention of long messages and inaccurate guessing by his partners. In addition, a busy nursing staff needed to spend several minutes to understand even the shortest messages. Furthermore, the approach was sufficiently complicated that unfamiliar partners could not communicate with Steve until they had received some training.

Future Needs. Steve expressed the desire to work toward two major goals: speaking and writing. In light of Steve's profound physical disability which would prevent him from taking an active part in so many of the activities that he had previously enjoyed, the staff agreed that the goal of normal speech was an extremely important one. Normal speech, a marvelously rapid, efficient communication system, would allow Steve to take part in social activities in ways that any less efficient systems would not.

Capability Assessment

Speech. At the time of our initial evaluation, tongue swelling continued to be a major obstacle in the production of precise articulatory movements. However, the swelling decreased somewhat when Steve's head was supported by pillows in an increasingly upright position. This permitted trials with an electrolarynx, which communication partners could activate for him.

Language and Cognition. Little formal language or cognitive testing was done initially because of Steve's limited communicative output and his inability to tolerate extended testing. We made informal observations of his ability to follow directions, to answer questions, and to generate messages using the extremely slow eye-gaze system. These suggested that language, memory, and intellectual abilities would not be limiting factors in selection of a communication or writing systems.

Motor Control. Steve's motor control abilities were consistent with a C1-2 spinal cord injury. He had no movement in any of his extremities and poor head control. His diaphragm was paralyzed bilaterally.

INTERVENTION

Phase I. Moving Toward Independent Speech

The Electrolarynx. The first phase of intervention had two goals: increasing the efficiency of communication and increasing Steve's communicative independence. This was accomplished in a series of steps. The first was to move from the slow eye-gaze system to more rapid speech with a partner-activated electrolarynx. We tried two types of electrolarynges. The first was a Cooper-Rand intraoral type (Fig. 6–3). Use of this system requires that a small plastic tube be positioned on the tongue. The speaker then produces exaggerated oral articulatory movements simultaneously with the activation of the tone generator. This system was our first choice because it could be adapted to permit activation by means of an eyebrow switch, thus allowing independent use. Unfortunately, Steve's swollen tongue interfered with his ability to tolerate the tube while maintaining precise articulation.

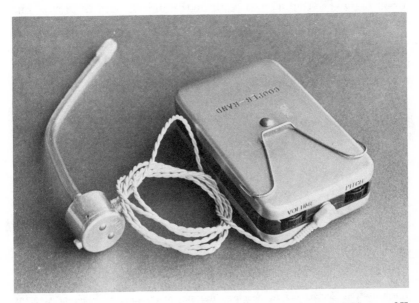

Figure 6–3. A Cooper-Rand electrolarynx, manufactured by Luminaud, Mentor, OH.

Our second choice was a neck type electrolarynx (Fig. 6-4), which was placed in contact with Steve's neck and activated by the communication partner. Simultaneously with his partner's activation, Steve would begin to articulate. With some practice to train overarticulation, Steve was able to communicate understandably. He found that communication with the electrolarynx was much more rapid and less fatiguing than the eye-gaze system. However, he remained frustrated by the lack of independence and the fact that only selected partners could effectively use the system with him. Some listeners had difficulty understanding Steve's speech. Others had difficulty in placing the electrolarynx properly and in coordinating its activation with the initiation of speech attempts.

Tracheostomy Cuff Deflation. The second phase of speech intervention involved attempts to route ventilatory air through the vocal folds so that Steve could achieve phonation. A cuff deflation procedure is illustrated in Figure 6-2 (right). During the insufflatory phase of the respirator's cycle, this procedure allows air to be routed up through the larynx as well as into the lungs. Once Steve's respiratory support and other medical problems had stabilized, a team including respiratory disease physicians, physiatrists, respiratory therapists, nurses, and speech-language pathologists worked together to formulate the following approach, which would allow Steve to speak. Prior to speaking trials, Steve's tracheostomy cuff would be deflated. Simultaneously, he was bagged so that a burst of air up through the larynx allowed him to swallow the secretions that had collected above the inflated cuff.

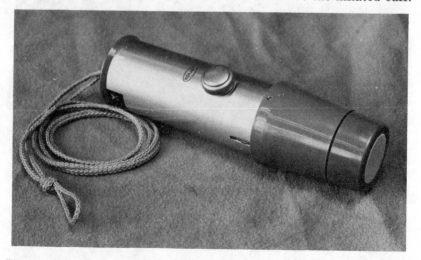

Figure 6-4. A Servox neck-type electrolarynx, distributed by Siemens Hearing Instruments, Inc., Union, NJ.

The respirator was adjusted to meet his ventilatory needs in the presence of a deflated cuff. Initially, Steve tolerated the cuff deflation for only about 10 minutes before he began to feel "short of air." His tolerance quickly increased to more extended period of time. Steve learned to coordinate speech attempts with the insufflation phase of the respirator. Within a few 10 minute training sessions, Steve could speak functionally. Steve easily learned to speak only on insufflation and to pause during exhalation.

To eliminate the flow of air through the larynx when Steve did not wish to speak, he was taught to adduct his vocal cords voluntarily. Initially, this training was accomplished by having him phonate briefly and then forcibly terminate phonation with an unreleased glottal stop. The cessation of phonation served as feedback to Steve that his vocal folds were forcibly adduced. After a few trials Steve was proficient at adducting his folds with the phonation technique. This maneuver eliminated the discomfort of air passing through the larynx and oral cavity when he was not speaking. It became so automatic that Steve was able to sleep with the vocal folds in the adducted position. Eventually, the cuff was deflated at all times, even when Steve was eating or sleeping.

Phrenic Nerve Pacing. Eventually bilateral phrenic nerve pacers were implanted surgically. These served to stimulate the nerve to his diaphragm so that he could be free from the respirator for extended periods of the day. In order to increase the amount of time Steve could be free of the respirator, he was paced on only one side of the diaphragm at a time while the other side was rested.

The Voice Amplifier. The intensity of Steve's voice was considerably reduced during unilateral pacing over that produce during bilateral pacing or respirator supported speech. With unilateral pacing, his voice was sufficiently loud to be understood in a face-to-face conversation in a quiet room, but he experienced difficulty when calling to someone in the next room or on occasion when talking on the telephone. A small, pocket-sized, battery-powered voice amplifier was given a trial (Fig. 6-5). Steve used it along with an eyeglass mounted microphone. The nursing staff believed that the amplifier worked well. When Steve used it, they were now able to move about the room and did not need to be continually in visual contact. Steve agreed that the amplifier made his speech louder and easier to understand. However, he operated his wheelchair with a sip-and-puff control and changed channels on the wheelchair with a chin lever. Therefore, he was not enthusiastic about still another device (the microphone) in proximity to his face. He chose to postpone the decision about purchasing the speech amplifier until he went home and could determine whether or not he needed one there.

Phase II. Writing System

The second major goal of our intervention was to develop a writing system. By this time in his rehabilitation, Steve had become proficient with the sip-and-puff interface that he used to drive his wheelchair. The writing system of choice for him was an Apple II + computer with the Adaptive Firmware Card. This writing system is similar to the one described for Keith in Chapter 3. The system was selected for several reasons. The first was the potential for use of the sip-and-puff interface with such a system. The second was that Steve had demonstrated sufficient ability to learn new material, and we were confident that he would easily and quickly learn Morse code. The third was the fact that the Adaptive Firmware Card emulates the Apple computer keyboard. Thus, Steve would have access to to wide variety of educational, business, recreational, and word processing software.

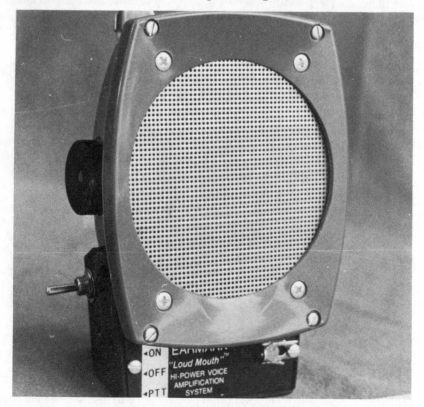

Figure 6-5. A portable voice amplifier.

Morse Code Training. Training was begun during a period when Steve was confined to bed for an extended period of time. Thus, training was begun using the A-Tronix keyer and sip-and-puff interface discussed in Chapter 3. This system is compact, is lightweight, and could be placed on a hospital table over Steve's bed so that he could practice while resting. He appeared to enjoy the break in his routine that this training afforded him.

Steve used the visual mnemonic system described in Chapter 3 during the initial phase of learning. A list of words that could be spelled in their entirety with letters that had been learned previously was provided after each training session. Thus, Steve began practicing on whole words as soon as he had learned only five letters. We encouraged him to send Morse code on a word-by-word rather than letter-by-letter basis, in order to avoid the motor control habits that initially reduced Keith's efficiency (see Chapter 3). Five new letters were added at each training session. Steve learned rapidly. Within 10 training sessions, he could accurately code the entire alphabet and a number of punctuation marks from memory. At this point, he began to explore a number of recreational software programs and to write letters using the word processing software. Steve's formal training did not proceed beyond this point. His rate of production of Morse code was slow, just under 8 words/minute. But he felt that it was adequate for his almost exclusively recreational purposes. If he had had immediate vocational plans or had the need to produce large amounts of text, more training to increase rate may have been considered.

QUESTIONS FOR THE CLINICIAN

Question 1. What are the problems of an electrolarynx held and operated by the communication partner? Are there any alternatives?

An electrolarynx is a device that provides a sound source for speech in those who cannot produce a voice. Depending on the type of electrolarynx, the sound source can be released in the mouth (as in the intraoral Cooper-Rand electrolarynx) or against the neck. The Servox, Aurex, and Western Electric types are among the commercially available neck-type electrolarynges. A user with good hand function operates the tone generation switch in synchrony with speech. The tone or voice is turned on precisely when the speaker wishes to initiate a phrase and is turned off immediately as the phrase is ended or when the speaker wishes to pause. Users without good hand function must rely on the partner for activation and release of the tone generator. Coordination between the speaker and communication partner takes a good deal of practice, and failure to coordinate the efforts results in speech that is very difficult to understand. Several electrolarynx users who were dependent on their communication partners for placement and activation of the device have complained to me of the problems caused by the lack of independent control. Some indicated that they were not easily able to get their partner's attention and thus were forced to rely on partners to initiate interactions. Others complained of just the opposite problem. At times, their communication partners would position the electrolarynx and activate the tone when the user did not wish to say anything. Steve indicated that he always felt obliged to say something when his partner would start his "voice."

A number of alternatives are becoming available for those who do not have sufficient hand function to hold the electrolarynx or to operate the tone generator manually. As was mentioned earlier in this chapter, the Cooper-Rand electrolarynx can be adapted for use with an eyebrow switch. A remotely controlled neck-type electrolarynx has been developed (Hammond, Cox, and Scarpelli, 1982).

At our center, a Cooper-Rand electrolarynx was modified to permit independent use by patients like Steve. As you can see in Figure 6-6, the modifications were simple. First, it was altered to permit remote activation. To this end, a plastic ring was used to hold the activation button in the "on" position. A circuit interrupter with a remote switch was placed on the circuit in such a way that the activation switch bypassed the interrupter and allowed the activation of the device. The remote control could be nearly any type of switch; we show it here with a head switch.

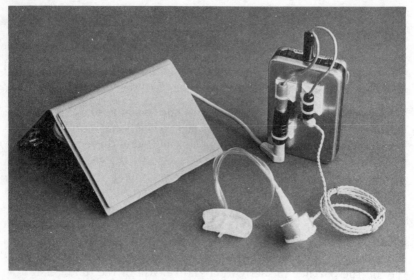

Figure 6-6. A remote control switch for the Cooper-Rand electrolarynx.

The second modification was made to the oral tube to provide for independent support in the mouth. The tube was replaced with a considerably longer tube. A rough dental impression was made of two or three of the user's teeth on the right or left and a hole was made in the impression to accommodate the oral tube. When the dental mold was affixed to the teeth by means of denture adhesive, the tube was supported in the proper place.

Question 2. Obviously, Steve's writing system was not portable. How do you decide when a writing system needs to be portable? What are the options for a portable Morse code–based writing system?

Decisions about portability of writing systems are made on the basis of the communication needs assessment. In Steve's case, a portable system would have been desirable but not mandatory. His discharge plans involved living in a small rural community. He planned to use the system at home and had no plans in the immediate future to extend its use to vocational activities outside the home. The computer-based writing system also has advantages in that Steve could use it for a variety of other functions, including recreational and household management activities.

Currently, there are two options for using the Epson HX-20 computer as a portable, Morse code–activated writing device. Adaptive Peripherals provides the translation with a keyboard emulator chip placed in the memory expansion module of the Epson HX-20.

Question 3. Have you generally been successful in reestablishing speech in respirator-dependent patients with limited hand control?

The staff of our center completed an 18 month survey of applications of augmentative communication systems for respirator-dependent patients (Beukelman, Yorkston, Dowden, Mitsuda, and Lossing, submitted for publication). We retrospectively gathered general information about the parients' medical histories, communication problems, communication needs, and systems that were recommended for their use. Our data base also included indication of the success or failure of the system to meet communication needs. The 19 cases included in our survey fell into three general groups. The first of these groups included patients who had intact cognitive abilities and had unrestricted control of the laryngeal and articulatory mechanism. As short-term communication solutions, the electrolarynx provided these patients with speech. Long-term communication alternatives for patients in this group included writing with a Morse code–based computer system and speaking with a deflated cuff. The second group of respirator-dependent patients whom we were able to serve were those with intact cognitive and language skills but restricted control of the oral speech mechanism. A number of communication augmentation systems provided these individuals with an alternative to speech. Our attempts to serve the third group of patients, respirator-dependent patients with severe cognitive or linguistic limitations, or both, were largely unsuccessful.

ACKNOWLEDGMENTS

Steve's stay at our hospital lasted several months, and therefore a number of individuals need to be acknowledged along with the entire rehabilitation team. Among these individuals are Laura Shillam, OTR, who was primarily responsible for the Morse code training for the computer-based writing system, Jan Trask, RN, Steve's primary nurse, and Diana Cardenas, MD, his attending physician.

REFERENCES

Beukelman, D. R., Yorkston, K. M., Dowden, P. A., Mitsuda, P., and Lossing, C. Communication augmentation applications with respirator-dependent patients. Submitted for publication.
Hammond, M. R., Cox, P. M., and Scarpelli, A. A remotely controlled neck-type electrolarynx for the tracheostomized quadriplegic. *ASHA*, 1982, *24*, 742.

ADDITIONAL READINGS

Donovan, W. H. Spinal cord injury. In W. C. Stolov and M. R. Clowers (Eds.), *Handbook of severe disability*. Washington, DC: US Department of Education, Rehabilitation Services Administration, 1981, pp. 65–82.
Sunners, J. The use of the electrolarynx in patients with temporary tracheostomies. *Journal of Speech and Hearing Disorders*, 1973, *38*, 335–338.

CHAPTER 7

Mark

Etiology: Amyotrophic lateral sclerosis (ALS)
Onset: 38 years of age
Approach: Living Center System on a TRS-80 Computer
Focus: This chapter describes the selection of a communication augmentation system for a man with a progressive neurologic disorder. His motor impairment, which limited him to the use of a single switch activated by head movements, was further complicated by reduced endurance. A computer-based scanning system with a large retrievable vocabulary was selected.

BACKGROUND

Mark's wife called our center for assistance when her husband was no longer able to communicate effectively with their two daughters. Only his wife was able to understand his speech, but she reported increasing difficulty. The couple was experiencing more and more unresolved communication breakdowns. It had been 18 months since Mark had received the formal diagnosis of amyotrophic lateral sclerosis (ALS). During the following months, this 38 year old teacher resigned his position and was confined to bed, wheelchair, or easy chair owing to weakness. No longer able to feed, dress, or toilet himself, Mark gradually became dependent upon his family to meet his daily needs. Throughout the early months he continued to communicate easily with his family, direct his physical care, assist his children with homework, and visit with friends. However, progressive dysarthria reduced Mark's ability to communicate with friends and attendants who came into the home to relieve his wife of her 24 hour responsibility for him.

Following his diagnosis, Mark learned a great deal about ALS. This progressive neurologic disease affects the nuclei of the motor nerves of the spinal and cranial systems. Both upper and lower motor neurons may be affected; therefore, spasticity as well as weakness may be an early symptom of the disease. Eventually extreme weakness and inability to move are the predominant symptoms. In Mark's case, the spinal nerves were affected earlier than the cranial nerves. Therefore, he experienced weakness in the arms and legs much earlier than in the throat and mouth, and he could speak and swallow long after he lost the ability to move about physically.

Mark's only remaining communication approach at the beginning of our intervention consisted of severely dysarthric speech and a very well trained primary communication partner, his wife. During the initial evaluation, his wife acted as an interpreter for Mark, because we were able to understand only 20% of his messages. When his wife failed to understand, he attempted to spell words aloud. Approximately 10% to 15% of the time, even his wife could not resolve communication breakdowns.

EVALUATION

Needs Assessment

Mark's communication needs list (Table 7–1) is adapted from the one that appears in Appendix I. The needs assessment was completed by Mark and his wife with assistance from the speech-language pathologist. It was determined that communication in bed and in Mark's easy chair were mandatory needs, while communication in the wheelchair was desired but not mandatory. Mark's physical limitations were such that he traveled minimally outside of his home, and he reported that he did not intend to change this pattern. He wished to have a communication system that would be sufficiently portable to be transported to the hospital, if necessary. His wife noted that she had remained with him the entire time during his previous hospitalization to act as an interpreter.

Mark felt that his primary communication need was to interact with his wife and children without communication failure. An additional mandatory need was to communicate with friends and attendants without requiring that his wife act as interpreter. Although Mark and his wife had not considered the ability to communicate with someone across the room or in another room as important, they quickly added this need to the list when they learned that augmentative communication systems had this potential. Mark's wish to communicate about a broad range of unique topics is reflected in the extensive mandatory needs for a large variety of message types (Table 7–1). Mark also indicated his intention to write letters as well as to write about his experience with ALS.

Table 7-1. Mark's Communication Needs List

Positions:

    M   In bed—supine
    M   In bed—sitting
    M   In easy chair
    D   In wheelchair

Communication Partners:

    M   Someone unfamiliar with the system
    D   Someone across the room or in another room
    D   Several people at a time
    M   Someone who can read

Locations:

    M   Bedroom (bed)
    M   Living room (easy chair)
    D   Kitchen (wheelchair)
    M   Hospital (bed and wheelchair)

Message Needs:

    M   Call attention
    M   Signal emergencies
    M   Answer yes/no questions
    M   Provide unique information
    M   Make requests
    M   Carry on a conversation
    M   Express emotion
    M   Give opinions
    M   Convey basic medical needs
    D   Greet people
    M   Prepare messages in advance
    D   Make notes
    D   Write letters

Key: M = Mandatory
      D = Desirable but not mandatory

Capability Assessment

Motor Control. The first question addressed in this motor control assessment was the following, "What movements could be used to control a system?" We completed a brief survey of various body parts. Mark was unable to move his legs, feet, or toes voluntarily. No movements at the elbow or wrist on his left side were observed. On the right side he demonstrated limited flexion and extension of the elbow but no movement of the wrist and fingers. He could activate the switch by "tossing" his right hand toward it using elbow flexion and extension, but he was unable to release and reactivate the switch promptly in this position. Therefore, use of his hand to activate a system was not considered. Mark was able to activate, release, and reactivate a momentary switch by elevating his right shoulder. However, we eliminated this movement from control options because of the progressive nature of his motor control impairment. We were not certain how much longer he would be able to move his shoulder.

With most of the other control options eliminated, we next considered head movements. Mark usually sat with his head resting against the headrest of an easy chair or supported in bed with a pillow. The chair provided lateral support to his trunk. He was able to flex at the shoulders, lift his head from the headrest to look around, and position his head for swallowing. He was also able to rotate his head from side to side while it was positioned against the headrest. Movement of his eyes and eyebrows appeared only minimally impaired. By the time the motor control assessment was completed, we had determined that head movements of some kind would be sufficient to control a communication augmentation system.

Head Control Options.   The next step in the motor assessment was to decide what type of system Mark would be able to control via the head movements we had identified. Our first choice would be a direct selection system, since this would give him the potential for a more rapid rate than would a scanning system. To evaluate Mark's ability to access a direct selection system using head movements, we used a Frameworks headlight pointer with an alphabet board. If he had demonstrated the ability to select letters on the alphabet board using this system, a more sophisticated, head-controlled direct selection system, such as the Express system (see Chapter 2) would have been given a trial. Unfortunately, after less than 1 minute of use, Mark reported neck fatigue and rejected this approach as a long-term motor control option. During the motor control assessment, Mark demonstrated the ability to operate a single switch positioned on either side of his head. He also demonstrated the control sequence of switch activation, release, and reactivation with the precision necessary to access a scanning communication system. Therefore, the capability assessment of motor control had narrowed our options to a head-controlled, scanning system.

Vision.   Mark and his wife reported no problems with his vision. He did not wear glasses. During our evaluation Mark demonstrated the ability to correctly identify letters on a computer screen positioned before him and on the computer printer.

Language.   Typically, language abilities are not affected in ALS. According to his wife, Mark was speaking in well-formed sentences with no evidence of difficulty in word finding or grammatical errors. During the initial portion of the evaluation, he verbally spelled the names of family members, doctors, medications, and locations without error. He also spelled phrases in attempts to resolve communication breakdowns. No formal spelling tests were administered because his spelling skills were judged to be adequate for a letter-by-letter approach to communication.

Cognition. Cognitive impairment is not usually associated with ALS. Early conversations with Mark revealed a man who was very aware of his situation. He discussed his communication needs and ideas about possible approaches to communication alternatives in a coherent and thoughtful manner. During the remainder of the evaluation, he demonstrated that he understood the functions of a variety of communication augmentation systems and learned to operate them quickly.

INTERVENTION

A Survey of Options

Our intervention program with Mark was completed in three phases. The first phase involved the education of Mark and his wife about communication options available to them. After reviewing various commercially available scanning systems, Mark and his wife decided to explore the computer-based systems in greater detail. They made this decision for two reasons. First, the computer offered a variety of communicative, recreational, and intellectual options that were not available in the dedicated communication systems. Second, Mark was interested in having a computer system available to his children when he was not using it.

Trials with the Systems

The second phase of intervention involved brief trials with two computer systems. The first was a system that we had assembled at our center for another client. This Apple computer-based system allowed the user to select words or phrases in their entirety using alphabetic and numeric codes with cues from the computer monitor. The system could be controlled through direct selection, scanning, or Morse code input. Output selections included screen display, speech synthesis, and print. During the trial, Mark demonstrated the ability to understand and control the system. Motorically, he accessed the system with a momentary switch positioned to the right of his head. The switch was activated by rotating his head while he rested it against the head support of an easy chair.

The second trial system was the Living Center System developed by Words +, Inc., Sunnyvale, California (Fig. 7-1). This system utilized a TRS-80 Radio Shack, Level 3, computer with specialized software, a computer printer, and a speech synthesizer. The Living Center program allows the user to retrieve complete words and phrases from a large dictionary of stored messages. The system has the capacity for a vocabulary of over 1300 words, supplemented with phrases. Sentences and phrases can be added or deleted by the user. Letter-by-letter message formulation is permitted. Words are retrieved by indicating the first letter of the word and then scanning through a string of words beginning with that letter until the preferred word is selected. Message output is accomplished through display on the screen, speech synthesis, or print. The Living Center System also contains functions other than communication, such as games, drawing, environmental control, and an alarm.

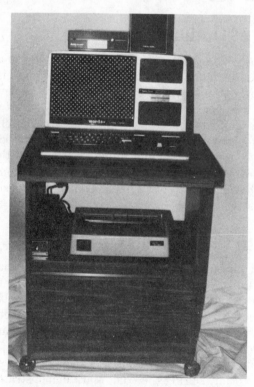

Figure 7-1. The Living Center System available from Words+, Inc., Sunnyvale, California.

Final Selection and Purchase

The third phase of Mark's intervention involved purchase of the Living Center. The family selected this system because they liked the greater breadth of vocabulary than was provided at that time by the system developed in our center. They were more comfortable with the TRS-80 computer, because Mark's wife had worked extensively with that equipment in her former teaching position. Because of Mark's urgent need for the communication equipment, he purchased it with personal funds. Simultaneously, a request was made to his medical insurance company, which was subsequently rejected. The Living Center equipment was mounted on a portable cart that could be moved from place to place in the home. A brow switch (Fig. 7-2) was selected as the interface of choice. Use of a switch positioned beside Mark's head was abandoned because of the difficulty in positioning it while Mark was in bed.

At the time this chapter was written, Mark was operating the Living Center system. It was meeting all of his mandatory and desired communication needs that were identified in the communication needs assessment. Besides facilitating communication, the computer has

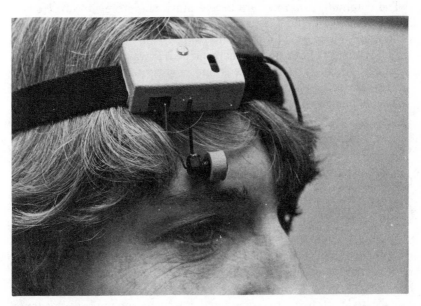

Figure 7-2. Mark's eyebrow switch with which he controlled the Living Center System.

provided an important point of contact between Mark and his children. In addition to communicating with them, he is able to play a selected set of games with them, and he has the obvious pleasure of observing his children enjoying the computer for recreation and educational activities.

COMMENTS FROM MARK'S WIFE

We had intended to ask Mark to comment on his communication system. However, his health deteriorated quite suddenly, and he died before we were able to do so. His wife supplied the following information.

"The Words + Living Center System allowed Mark to communicate specific words and phrases when I could not understand him. This was especially good when he wanted to ask doctors a specific question or describe a specific symptom. The system was a good conversation piece. Mark enjoyed demonstrating the system to friends. This often helped to ease their discomfort with his terminal disease . . . . Many friends were more willing to come by after they saw this system demonstrated. They felt it made Mark more comfortable, since he was able to communicate with them. In short, it helped remove the isolation factor when one has no speech."

The communication system "gave Mark something to do. He was actively involved—no longer just a spectator . . . . He could write out notes and messages to the kids and to me at his leisure." The transportability of the system really helped. It was taken to the hospital during the last visit. There was one negative aspect. The scanning approach was "not a comfortable mode of communication. Mark would get nervous after concentrating so hard."

QUESTIONS FOR THE CLINICIAN

Question 1. What is the difference between a computer-based communication augmentation system and a dedicated system? What are the considerations when selecting one over the other?

As the name implies, a computer-based communication augmentation system includes a computer for which software has been programmed to meet the communication needs of the user. Other educational, business, or recreational software can also be used with such a system. A dedicated system, on the other hand, may have computer components; however, its use is limited to the communication functions for which it was designed. Other software programs will not operate on a dedicated system.

There are several issues that must be explored when considering a computer-based versus a dedicated system. In Mark's case we carefully considered his present and long-term needs for a portable system. The Living Center system is hosted by a computer that requires wall power from a wall outlet and cannot be mounted on a wheelchair. However, it can be mounted on a cart with casters. Because Mark owned a van, we decided that his wife could move the system on the cart without disassembling it. A second issue is the availability of adequate software. In this application, the software package had been used by other individuals, and we were confident that Mark would not require the services of a computer programmer to implement the programs. Especially in the case of a patient with ALS, we are extremely reluctant to provide a system that will require extensive individualization. If the disease is rapidly progressive, the user might not have communication options available when they need them. A third consideration is the attitude of the family. Mark's family wanted a computer and had worked with computers previously. If they had been inexperienced or perhaps feared computers, we might have made a different decision.

Question 2. Do you serve an individual with degenerative disease differently from an individual with a stable or recovering condition?

Yes, management of individuals with degenerative disorders is different from the management of stable or recovering patients. As we indicated in the previous answer, a person with degenerative disease may not have the time for a long individualization or training phase. Therefore, we try to provide a system that works for them at the time of delivery. We also are very conservative in selecting systems to match the capability areas in which we expect deterioration. For example, in ALS we expect motor deterioration and select interface options that individuals can use both immediately and in the future, even if further deterioration occurs. If the condition is associated with progressive visual impairment, we select a system which can be used with a visual control display for the present, but perhaps can have an auditory control display added later. Possibly, we might select an approach like Morse code, for which no visual display is required. We also consider the ability of a family to use or to dispose of the equipment after the individual with degenerative disease no longer is able to use it. In some cases a standard unmodified computer or a commonly used communication augmentation aid will allow for profitable and rapid sale at a later time.

For some individuals, ALS is a rapidly progressive disease; some patients, however, live for 12 to 15 years following diagnosis (Sitver and Kraat, 1982). Sitver and Kraat followed 38 individuals with ALS who required communication augmentation. Review of their data revealed that 42% of their patients used a communication augmentation approach for 1 year or less. Several individuals used their systems for up to 6 years, and one person was still using the system after 12 years.

Question 3.   With an individual who is able to operate a single switch, how do you decide whether to select a scanning system or a system based on Morse code input?

There are several considerations. First, the visual requirements of scanning and Morse code control are quite different. The user memorizes Morse code, thus eliminating the need to observe a large array of message options and a traveling cursor or light, as is necessary with a scanning system.

Second, the motor control requirements also differ. In scanning, the user interrupts the activity of the system at precise times to indicate choices; however, during times when the switch is not activated, the user is at rest motorically. With the single switch Morse code approach, the user is motorically active almost continuously as the switch is activated, held, and released. For the individual who fatigues easily, Morse code control may be very tiring.

Third, single switch Morse code requires a high degree of motor timing, as the time relationship between dits, dahs, and pauses must be rigorously maintained. This requires a high level of control for activation, release, and reactivation of the switch. In interrupted scanning, the user must carefully time switch activation in order to interrupt the cursor pattern at the desired moment. In directed scanning, the user must carefully time switch release, in order to stop cursor movement. However, in neither interrupted nor directed scan are the timing requirements of the entire motor movement pattern as precise as in single switch Morse code control.

ACKNOWLEDGMENTS

We wish to acknowledge the assistance of Walter Waltosz of Words+, Inc., who promptly answered numerous questions about the Living Center System.

REFERENCES

Sitver, M. S., and Kraat, A. Augmentative communication for the person with amyotrophic lateral sclerosis (ALS). *ASHA*, 1982, *24*, 783.

ADDITIONAL READINGS

Adams, M. R. Communication aids for patients with amyotrophic lateral sclerosis. Journal of Speech and Hearing Disorders, 1966, *31*, 274–275.

Beukelman, D. R., and Yorkston, K. M. Computer enhancement of message formulation and presentation for communication augmentation system users. *Seminars in Speech and Language*, 1984, *5*, 1–10.

Johnson, E. N., and Alexander, M. A. Management of motor unit diseases. In F. Kottke, G. Stillwell, and J. Lehmann (Eds.), *Krusen's handbook of physical medicine and rehabilitation* (3rd Edition). Philadelphia, W. B. Saunders Co., 1982, pp. 679–690.

CHAPTER 8

Daniel

Etiology: Amyotrophic lateral sclerosis (ALS)
Onset: 55 years of age
Approach: Alphabet board for speech supplementation
               Sharp Memowriter
Focus: This is the case of a man with ALS who spoke but was difficult to understand. It was recommended that he use an alphabet supplementation approach to increase the intelligibility of his speech. A Sharp Memowriter was recommended as a portable writing system. We discuss the issue of the transition to augmentative systems for individuals with degenerative diseases.

BACKGROUND

Daniel is a 58 year old engineer who was employed until 1983 at the Boeing Company. From 1980 to September 1983, he was also the chairperson of the Seattle Transit Advisory Committee, an organization which makes recommendations to the mayor and his council about the city's transportation needs. In June of 1981, Daniel was diagnosed as having amyotrophic lateral sclerosis (ALS). As you know from the discussion in Chapter 7, this progressive neurologic disease takes several forms and is characterized by a variety of signs and symptoms. In Daniel's case, the disease was initially characterized by spasticity of the legs and flaccidity of the arms.

EVALUATION

Daniel was referred to our center in October 1983. He had a thorough understanding of his disease and its common courses, as well as a good grasp of what this would mean in his life. He wished to learn all about the equipment that might serve his needs now or in the future, so that he could make informed choices to meet these needs appropriately. It was always clear that Daniel had an unusually sophisticated approach to managing his own health care. He was his own best advocate and, given the proper information regarding communication augmentation, he would make his own decisions. In order to manage his communication problems, he wished to have a portable writing system and a means of augmenting his inconsistently intelligible speech.

At the time he came to our center, Daniel indicated that he used a wheelchair because of severe weakness in his legs. He indicated that he spent approximately one quarter of his day in the wheelchair or in his office chair at home. Half of his day was spent lying down. He walked short distances with a cane, but this was becoming considerably more difficult and fatiguing.

Capability Assessment

Motor Control.   Daniel's upper extremities were not symmetrically involved by the disease. He showed severe flaccidity of his nondominant left arm and hand, but only mild weakness of the right hand. He found that handwriting had become a laborious and exhausting process, with the results frequently illegible to others. Daniel showed sufficient fine motor control of his right hand to activate keys as small as 0.5 inch in diameter. He was able to depress such keys if the excursion and pressure required were not unusually great. This meant that he had sufficient motor control to use most of the commonly available keyboard devices, including the Deluxe Sharp Memowriter EL-7100, the Expanded Keyboard Sharp, the Canon Communicator, and the Epson HX-20 computer, as well as some standard electric typewriters and computer keyboards.

Vision.   Daniel showed sufficient visual acuity to read print as small as that produced with a standard typewriter. He was able to read the letters on all the keyboard devices already mentioned.

Speech and Language.   Daniel's speech was characterized by reduced loudness, insufficient breath support, hypernasality, and severe distortion of consonants due to reduced strength of the articulators. The result was poor intelligibility unless the context of the utterance was clear to the listener. His speech remained intelligible to his closest friends and family members, but communicating with strangers or business colleagues was extremely difficult. A close friend of the family had assumed the role of an aide as well as an interpreter for some occasions. Since ALS is not usually characterized by language deficits, we did no formal testing of Daniel's spelling or other language skills. Trials with the devices suggested that he had adequate language skills to communicate using a letter-by-letter message preparation approach.

Needs Assessment

Establishing Daniel's communication needs was relatively easy because of his insight into his disease and its course. He indicated that his current needs were limited. First, he wished to increase the intelligibility of his speech with listeners who were not familiar with him. Second, he needed a portable writing system for business purposes. From these general needs, we established a list of needs for the immediate future.

Daniel indicated that a speech augmentation system would have to do the following:

1. Increase his speech intelligibility with strangers to a more functional level.
2. Be intelligible to listeners who had not been specially trained.
3. Be portable and readily accessible.
4. Not decrease his communication rate substantially.

Daniel specified that the ideal writing system for him would have the following design characteristics:

1. Print letters of the alphabet as well as words and phrases.
2. Have keys at least 0.5 inch apart so that he could access them efficiently at this time and in the near future.
3. Have a keyguard that could support his hand on the device and prevent inadvertent activation of the keys.
4. Be flexible enough so that the device could be accessed by him in other ways as his motor control decreases.
5. Fit securely onto the armrest of his wheelchair.
6. Be small enough so as not to interfere with transfers into and out of the chair.
7. Have some memory capabilities so that he could make notes to himself or others and store them for later use.
8. Have enough memory capabilities so that letters and longer text could be stored for later completion.
9. Have hard copy printout.
10. Be battery operated with rechargeable batteries.
11. Be relatively inexpensive, since it was likely that Daniel would use the device only for a limited period of time.

RECOMMENDATIONS

Speech Supplementation

We recommended that he use an alphabet board (Fig. 8–1) for supplementation, pointing to the first letter of each word as he spoke the word (Beukelman and Yorkston, 1977). The immediate result was that we were able to converse with him without the aid of his interpreter. Communication breakdowns occurred, but they could be resolved by simple repetition or by Daniel's spelling the word on the board. His aide was able to understand him without breakdowns when Daniel used the supplementation approach described.

Daniel appreciated the importance of this approach for strangers. He felt that this would allow him to continue working and interacting with relatively unfamiliar people in an independent manner without an interpreter. This approach would allow him to continue speaking in situations in which he would have needed to write without the supplementation approach. Since the pace of a business meeting requires rapid communication, this approach would permit him to maintain an active rather than a peripheral role in discussions. Daniel seemed to show little or no reluctance to use the alphabet board in this manner. We recommended that he point to the letters on the keyboard of the Sharp instead of the alphabet board once the Memowriter had been mounted onto his wheelchair.

Writing System

Results of our evaluation suggested that at this time, Daniel was able to use most keyboard devices. It was important, therefore, to assess

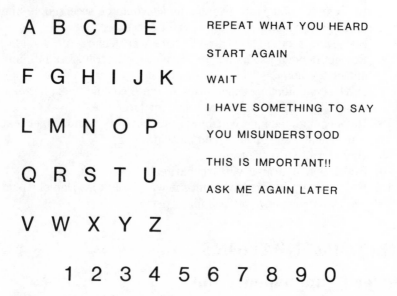

Figure 8-1. The alphabet phrase board used with the alphabet supplementation approach.

how well each device could meet the other needs described earlier. By working through the list it can be seen that some systems clearly did not meet his communication needs. For example, the requirement of portability was not met by a number of the systems, including personal computers and standard electric typewriters. The Sharp EL-7100, the Expanded Sharp, the Canon Communicator, and the Epson HX-20 computer were small enough that they could be mounted onto Daniel's wheelchair and not interfere with transfers. Each of these devices had the requisite hard copy print out and was operated with rechargable batteries. The Canon Communicator was eliminated from selection consideration because of the tape printout and lack of memory.

The major difference in the remaining systems is their relative power. The Epson HX-20 computer (Fig. 5–4) is clearly the most powerful in several respects. First, it has a memory capacity of 16K, expandable to 32K. Second, it comes equipped with a word processing chip, Skiwriter, and a microcassette storage system. This permits the user to store two or three documents on the cassette and load each document into the Epson for word processing. The third advantage is that the Epson HX-20 can print documents on its built-in tape printer as well as on a standard computer printer through an RS-232 cable. This permits the user to write formal documents on standard 8½ by 11 inch paper. The cost of the basic Epson HX-20 at this writing is approximately $800.

The Sharp Memowriters (the Sharp EL-7100 and the Expanded Keyboard Memowriters) shown in Figure 8–2 are considerably less powerful than the Epson HX-20 computer. They have some memory

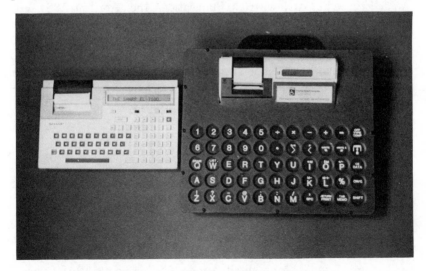

Figure 8–2. The Sharp Memowriters.

capacity in that up to 800 characters can be stored. However, there is no word processing capability beyond simple corrections and additions. The printout is limited to calculator-size paper type (Fig. 8–2) with 20 characters per line. At this time, the Sharp EL-7100 Memowriter costs approximately $200; the Expanded Keyboard model costs approximately $800. A keyguard for the Deluxe model is available through Zygo Industries, Inc. (Portland, OR), for approximately $100.

Daniel weighed all of these options and decided to use the Sharp EL-7100. He chose to forego the extra memory and printing capabilities of the Epson HX-20 computer because of the relative cost. He planned to look into dedicated communication devices with limited switch access when his motor control changed and the Sharp system ceased to meet his needs.

FOLLOW-UP

Eight months after this evaluation Daniel and his wife reported that he was still using the Sharp EL-7100 Memowriter. In the intervening months, his speech had become unintelligible even with the alphabet supplementation approach, and he had lost much of the use of his legs and left arm. He entered a nursing home, where he developed an elaborate system of multiple approaches to communication. He used the Sharp EL-7100 Memowriter, aided by a mobile arm support, for messages to the nursing staff regarding self-care. He used a standard typewriter for writing lengthy documents, such as an article published in *The Village Voice* (Newsgroup Publications, Inc., April 17, 1984, Vol. 29 [16], p. 1). He used the alphabet board for spelling in conversation with his wife or close friends. Some words and phrases were added to the board for more rapid delivery of predictable messages. He had also begun to use many one-handed gestures in communication with his wife. At the time this chapter was written, he had not yet decided to use a scanning communication approach.

QUESTIONS FOR THE CLINICIAN

Question 1. When do you typically intervene with treatment for individuals with a degenerative neuromotor speech disorder?

We intervene with these individuals at critical points during the course of their disease when their current approaches to communication do not meet their needs. Typically, the first point occurs when speech is no longer intelligible in all situations. At this point, a brief period of traditional speech treatment may be undertaken. This treatment may involve an effort to maximize intelligibility through rate control training or through prosthetic management, such as palatal lift fitting or the use of speech amplification. Of course, this treatment is based on the specific pattern of deficits seen in the individual. Another critical point of intervention may occur when speech is no longer functional, at least in some situations. At this time supplementation of speech or alternative communication must be considered. At both points, intervention is brief, whether it be more traditional speech training or the selection of a communication system. As we indicated in Chapter 7, we select systems that the individual is able to use without extensive training.

Question 2. When do you recommend that an individual with a degenerative speech disorder make the transition from speech to an alternative communication system?

Speech is such a wonderfully efficient and flexible means of communication that we attempt to find ways in which our patients can use speech as long as possible—i.e., as long as it serves their needs in some communication situations. The transition from speech to reliance on an alternative system is not an "all or nothing" process. A number of transitional steps, which may be called "limited speech," are useful in helping the individual to maximize residual speech abilities.

A number of different techniques fall under the heading of limited speech. The first is the alphabet supplementation approach recommended for Daniel and described in detail earlier. This approach allows individuals to use speech much longer in the course of their disease than they would without such supplementation.

A second type of limited speech involves the use of multiple approaches to communication. At times the approach used depends on the communicative function. Even the most severely dysarthric speakers can be understood if the communication situation is predictable enough. For example, many nearly unintelligible speakers continue to use speech for greetings and to answer yes or no questions. At times, the approaches depend on the communication partner. Some partners are simply better interpreters of severely dysarthric speech than others. Often the most successful communication partners are those who are the most familiar with the speaker's history, daily routine, communication style, and so forth. Table 8-1 contains a grid that summarizes the systems used by a severely dysarthric woman with ALS. She used three different approaches, depending on her communication partner and the message. She used speech in predictable communication situations, such as greetings or with the most familiar of her partners, her husband. She used speech supplemented with the alphabet on the keyboard of her Sharp Memowriter to communicate with her attendant and to resolve communication breakdowns with her husband. In difficult communication situations, where the accuracy of the output was critical and the messages unpredictable, she printed her messages on the Sharp Memowriter. She also used the Sharp Memowriter exclusively with unfamiliar partners, such as her nurse, who visited once a week.

Table 8-1. Approaches to Communication Used by a Woman with ALS for Different Communicative Functions and Communicative Partners

| | Partners | | |
	Husband	Attendant	Visiting Nurse
Greetings	Speech	Speech	Speech
Conversation	Speech	Speech supplemented with alphabet	Sharp Memowriter
Introducing new topic	Speech supplemented with alphabet	Speech supplemented with alphabet	Sharp Memowriter
Resolution of communication breakdown	Speech supplemented with alphabet	Sharp Memowriter	Sharp Memowriter

The third type of limited speech is used only with the most severely dysarthric speakers. This approach involves the use of a limited lexicon. At this point the speakers are usually using a communication augmentation system for the majority of their messages but are able to produce a few words understandably. A list of words and phrases that the speaker will attempt to produce verbally may be displayed on the wheelchair laptray or on the alphabet board. Such lists increase the potential for the partner to understand a highly distorted word or phrase by providing a "multiple choice selection." Often a word can be identified from a list of choices when it would not be understood if it were produced in isolation.

Question 3. For what types of patients do you recommend the alphabet supplementation approach? How do you train them to use it?

There are two broad categories of speakers who appear to benefit from the alphabet supplementation approach. Both types of speakers are so severely impaired that they are not able to speak understandably without supplementation. The first group of speakers are those whose speaking rate is more rapid than their level of motor control and coordination will support. Included in this category are many patients with Parkinson's disease and those with an ataxic speech pattern characterized by poor coordination of the complex series of movements required for speech. The second group of patients who benefit from the alphabet supplementation system includes those with such imprecise articulatory movements that they are not understood by their partners. This pattern of deficits is typical of individuals with severe flaccid or spastic dysarthria.

The alphabet supplementation approach appears to serve a different function with each of these speaker groups. For the first group, speaking rate is slowed as the speaker finds the desired letter and points to it. When the alphabet supplementation system is used in this way, as a pacing system, the communication partner may not actually need to see the alphabet letter indicated by the speaker. For the second group of speakers, it is critical that the communication partner see each letter. The supplementation approach works for this group because it provides the listener with extra information, which is necessary to enhance intelligibility. Daniel and most other individuals with ALS fall into the second group.

Training of the patient to use the system is fairly straightforward, especially with a cognitively intact individual. After the dysarthric individuals learn the mechanics of the speaking-pointing task, we begin to train them to manage their communication partners during conversational interactions. We recommend that users of an alphabet supplementation approach write instructions and mount them on the back of the alphabet board. Table 8–2 contains an example of the instructions that one patient chose to use. The written instructions can be used either to familiarize new communication partners or to reinstruct partners who are not following the rules of exchange.

Many alphabet boards contain not only the alphabet and numbers but also some conversational control phrases. These serve to remind the partner about the rules of exchange. For example, some severely dysarthric speakers use the word "Repeat" to remind their partners to say every word after them. This is quite unnatural for some communication partners, who would prefer to wait until the end of the entire sentence before repeating it. Unfortunately, if partners wait until the end of the sentence before repeating, communication breakdowns are more difficult to resolve. A number of proficient users of the alphabet supplementation approach have expressed their frustration with partners who repeat only at the end of sentences but have failed to understand one of the initial words of the sentence. When this

Table 8–2. Instructions Appearing on the Back of an Alphabet Supplementation Board of a Severely Dysarthric Speaker

I will point to the first letter of each word as I say that word.

Please repeat each word after me as I say it.

If you are right, I'll go on to the next word.

If you are wrong, I'll spell out the whole word for you.

I'll let you know when I'm finished with a sentence by pointing to "END OF SENTENCE."

happens, the dysarthric speaker needs to say almost the entire sentence over again to resolve the breakdown. If the partner had repeated word by word, resolution of the breakdown frequently would have required only a single word repetition or spelling. Other phrases on alphabet boards serve to maintain conversational control. For example, they may be used to initiate exchanges, such as "I have something to tell you." Other phrases serve to maintain conversational turns, for example, "Wait." Although we often recommend that some system users be telegraphic, we encourage those who use an alphabet supplementation approach to produce grammatically complete utterances. These utterances add redundancy to the message and therefore serve to increase its intelligibility.

Question 4.   You indicated at the time you assessed Daniel and made your recommendations to him that the Epson HX-20 could only be operated as a direct selection system. Is this still the case? If not, what are the current interface options available for the Epson?

Morse code is now feasible with the Epson HX-20. There are two ways in which a user can access the Epson with Morse code designed by two companies. Words +, Inc., sells a software program on cassette which, once loaded into the Epson, permits the user to activate single or double switches for Morse code. At this time, the program does not permit the user complete independence in loading and setting up the Morse code program. Paul Schwejda of Adaptive Peripherals developed a keyboard emulator, which is inserted into the memory expansion unit of the Epson HX-20 computer. The keyboard emulator allows two switch Morse code control of the computer and is transparent to most Epson software, to make a keyboard emulator for the Epson. At this time, the Trace Center (Madison, WI) is developing software for the Epson HX-20. The Trace Center plans the following functional modules: (1) simple text editor, (2) direct output to external voice, (3) keyboard emulation via Morse code or scanning, (4) calculator functions, and (5) abbreviation expansion (message retrieval).

REFERENCES

Beukelman, D. R., and Yorkston, K. M. A communication system for severely dysarthric individuals with an intact language system. *Journal of Speech and Hearing Disorders,* 1977, *42,* 265–270.

ADDITIONAL READINGS

Adams, M. R. Communication aids for patients with amyotrophic lateral sclerosis. *Journal of Speech and Hearing Disorders,* 1966, *31,* 274–275.

Beukelman, D. R., Yorkston, K. M. Gorhoff, S.C., Mitsuda, P. M., and Kenyon, V. T. Canon Communicator use by adults: A retrospective study. *Journal of Speech and Hearing Disorders,* 1981, *46,* 374–378.

Darley, F. L., Aronson, A. E., and Brown, J. R. *Motor speech disorders.* Philadelphia: W.B. Saunders, 1975.

Johnson, E. W., and Alexander, M. A. Management of motor unit diseases. In F. Kottke, G. Stillwell, and J. Lehmann (Eds.), *Krusen's Handbook of Physical Medicine and Rehabilitation* (pp. 679–690). Philadelphia: W.B. Saunders, 1982.

Rosenbek, J. C., and LaPointe, L. L. Dysarthria: Description, diagnosis and treatment. In D. F. Johns (Ed.), *Clinical management of neurogenic communication disorders.* Boston: Little, Brown & Company, 1978.

CHAPTER 9

Charlie

Etiology: Total laryngectomy; total glossectomy
Onset: 54 years of age
Approach: Gestures and a communication book
Focus: This chapter describes the case of a nonreading man who was unable to speak following a total laryngectomy and total glossectomy. A multi-modality approach to communication is described involving several applications of gestural and communication book approaches. We discuss the issues of lexicon selection and training patients and families in multiple system use.

BACKGROUND

Charlie is a 54 year old man who underwent a total laryngectomy with left radical neck dissection for laryngeal cancer in early 1983. Following this surgery, he became a functional user of an electrolarynx until the recurrence of cancer necessitated additional surgery. Six months later he underwent a total glossectomy with a right radical neck dissection.

Prior to the second surgery, Charlie was living with his sister in another state, where he had retired from farming. His sons and daughters lived in scattered areas of the United States. It was decided that he would come to Seattle for the surgery because one of his sons was stationed nearby. Because Charlie had been self-employed, funding remained a serious problem, although Medicaid funded his hospital stay.

Charlie's background was notable in that he had not learned to read or write more than the most rudimentary words. The reading skills of his primary caregiver, his sister, were functional but also limited.

INITIAL EVALUATION

Capability Assessment

Motor Control. Charlie was referred to our center for communication augmentation shortly after his glossectomy. At the time of the initial evaluation, he was alert and oriented and followed all commands. He was confined to bed and had significant pain upon movement of the right shoulder because of the pectoral flaps. For these reasons, all testing was limited to screening, and no evaluation of writing ability was attempted at this time.

Vision and Hearing.   Assessment of Charlie's visual abilities was limited by his poor reading skills and by the shoulder pain, which precluded his copying drawings or shapes. However, his visual abilities appeared to be within normal limits. He showed a mild to moderate hearing loss in the left ear but unimpaired hearing in the right ear.

Language and Cognition.   Charlie's reading abilities were screened with phrase and word recognition tasks. The results indicated that he had virtually no reading recognition except for digits, names of family members, and very commonplace names. Charlie's spelling level could not be assessed at this time. Later evaluation showed that he could spell few words, although he knew the first letter of some place names (e.g., "C" for California) and of some family members' names.

Communication Needs Assessment

Before goals and approaches to therapy could be planned, it was necessary to determine Charlie's communication needs for the postoperative phase as well as for his return home. This required patient and family interviews concerning his home environment, habits, and interests, as well as the interests and abilities of his family members. As part of this interview a needs assessment questionnaire was completed, and the following general needs were discussed.

Regarding Environment.   Charlie needed to communicate at home as well as in other locations (e.g., in friends' homes, in stores, while walking). He wanted to communicate over the telephone with his family, and, in times of emergency, with strangers. This meant that Charlie's communication systems would have to be portable and provide him with a means of using the telephone.

Regarding Partners.   Any system for Charlie would have to be understandable to individuals with little or no reading ability. The system would have to be useful even with individuals who were unfamiliar with it, such as store clerks. In addition, Charlie would be communicating with more than one person at a time and with individuals who had a limited amount of time on some occasions.

Regarding Message Needs. Charlie would need to talk about an unlimited number of topics. It should be noted, however, that because he was physically able to care for himself, he had essentially no need to make basic requests such as "I need some water." Instead, he would need to discuss more abstract and less easily predictable concepts. The patient would also need to use language in an unlimited number of ways. For example, he would need to give information as well as ask questions, signal and correct misunderstandings, call attention, signal and describe emergencies, make requests, and so on.

From this general information we were able to formulate specific communication needs for Charlie. Table 9–1 lists these needs in detail.

INTERVENTION

Selection of Approaches

Charlie was clearly not easy to serve using conventional approaches to communication augmentation. His poor spelling and reading recognition precluded the primary use of systems with letter or word displays. His picture recognition skills were good, but the use of picture or symbol displays would greatly limit the number of topics he could express with most systems. Because Charlie was able to walk and could care for most of his own needs, he would have little need to convey many of the simple picturable concepts, such as "thirsty" or "hungry."

Funding was an additional complicating factor in that Charlie had received the funds to remain in this hospital for only a few weeks. It was presumed that at the end of his hospitalization, he would return to his home state. This precluded teaching Charlie the use of an elaborate encoded approach with speech output, such as the Minspeak described in Chapter 2. Furthermore, the patient and his family rejected any devices with speech output (for example, the Vocaid) as too unnatural.

Charlie and his family preferred to use what they considered more "natural" forms of communication: gestures and a communication book. These approaches were actually a combination of communication techniques we taught Charlie.

Gestural Approaches

Symbolic Gestures. These gestures, based on Skelly's (1979) American Indian Sign Language (Amer-Ind), were used to express concrete and referential concepts. As we describe below, we began teaching Skelly's gestures but found that we could be more successful

Table 9-1. Specific Needs Statements for Charlie

Positioning

In bed

    M   In a variety of positions

Related to mobility:

    M   Must carry the system while walking

Communication Partners

    M   Someone who cannot read (e.g. child or non-reader)
    M   Someone with no familiarity with the system
    D   Someone who is across the room or in another room
    M   Several people at a time
    M   Someone who has limited time

Locations

    M   In multiple rooms within the same building
    M   In several buildings
    M   While moving from place to place within a building
    M   In dimly lit rooms
    M   In bright rooms
    M   In noisy rooms
    M   Outdoors
    M   While traveling in a car, van, and so forth
    M   In more than two locations
    M   In friends' homes
    M   In stores

Message Needs

    M   Call attention
    M   Signal emergencies
    M   Answer yes/no questions
    M   Provide unique information
    M   Make requests
    M   Carry on a conversation
    M   Express emotion
    M   Give opinions
    M   Convey basic medical needs
    M   Greet people

Modality Of Communication

    M   Talk on the phone in emergencies
    D   Converse on the phone

Key: M = Mandatory

      D = Desirable but not mandatory

if we elicited Charlie's spontaneous gestures and then modified them according to Skelly's principles. This strategy proved necessary because we saw the strong influence of culture on Charlie's choice of gestures and on his family's comprehension.

Tracing Symbols. Charlie utilized tracing in the palm of his hand, in the air, or on a table top for some concepts. For example, single or double digit numbers as well as the first letter of family members' names were easily conveyed in this manner.

Drawing. Some complex concepts were best expressed by Charlie's drawing, e.g., the cornfields on his farm.

Facial Expressions. Charlie used exaggerated facial expressions to convey emotions such as puzzlement, confusion, anger, and so forth.

Mouthing Words. Charlie was able to mouthe some words. This became an effective means of conveying a select number of words that could be lipread easily. Because of his total glossectomy, he would probably not be able to use the electrolarynx much more effectively than he could mouth words. Either approach would most likely be used only for vocabulary with highly "visible" phonemes, such as the bilabial sounds in "'Pam," the name of his primary nurse.

Communication Book Approaches

Written Words with Line Drawings. A book was designed with simple line drawings, to cue Charlie, paired with written words for the listener. The items included in the book were concepts which could not be gestured easily, such as "surgery," "adhesive tape," "gauze," and so forth. Line drawings were chosen to serve as cues in word recognition for Charlie or for nonreading listeners. Some examples of these entries appear in Figure 9-1.

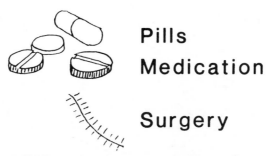

Pills

Medication

Surgery

FIGURE 9-1. Words coupled with line drawings.

Line Drawings.   These were used in the communication book without accompanying words for items that were best shown visually, such as a clock face for indicating time and a calendar for indicating days and months (Fig. 9–2).

Emergency Communication

A cassette tape recorder was recommended for use over the telephone in case of emergency. Prerecorded messages were made to summon a police car, an ambulance, or a firetruck.

Of the foregoing approaches, Charlie relied most heavily on the gestural techniques. He usually conveyed his messages with facial expressions, gestures, tracing in the palm of his hand, and mouthing words. If necessary, he would "resort" to drawing or the use of the word book.

Training

Basic Gestures.   In the first week of training we had essentially two goals. First, Charlie needed immediately a means of conveying basic medical concepts for his daily care. Second, he needed to understand the use of multiple approaches to communication. We intended to teach him enough of each approach to meet these basic needs. Initially, this would allow him to meet some needs by gesturing and other needs by means of a rudimentary communication book.

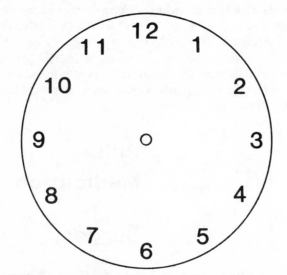

FIGURE 9–2. Line drawings used without written words.

Charlie was seen daily for training in these approaches, except when other procedures prohibited. Therapy was designed along the lines of the approach developed for aphasic individuals, called Promoting Aphasic Communicative Effectiveness (PACE), (Davis and Wilcox, 1981). In order to simulate natural conversation, there had to be one communication partner who had no prior knowledge of the content of the messages to be conveyed. Because Charlie could not read written stimuli and we were working in complex concepts that could not always be represented in pictures, we utilized a student clinician in the role of uninformed listener. The primary clinician provided the stimuli for each drill, and the student determined whether Charlie's efforts were intelligible, by attempting to interpret his messages.

Throughout the early sessions, when his condition was medically unstable, Charlie had some difficulty imitating gestures; rapid acquisition of any new gestures seemed virtually impossible. However, Charlie's spontaneous gestures were quite rich and clear, so we began by compiling a record of them. We asked the staff to keep a diary of his gestures and we found that he often had more than one gesture for the same concept. For this reason, our first goal was to teach Charlie which of his spontaneous gestures to rely upon, which to abandon. By the end of the second week, Charlie had a repertoire of some 85 reliable gestures. Table 9-2 provides excerpts from the diary kept by the hospital staff.

Table 9-2. Spontaneous Gesture Diary

Date	Idea Charlie Conveyed	How He Conveyed It or How You Understood It
2/12/83	I'm hungry	He pointed to his mouth and patted his stomach
2/12/83	When can I eat real food?	Pointed to his mouth; shrugged his shoulders; pretended to take out nasogastric tube
2/12/83	When can I go home?	Pointed to calendar; nurse asked yes/no questions

In this phase of intervention, we made a rudimentary word and line-drawing book (Figs. 9-1 and 9-2). Just as for the gestures above, we relied on Charlie's spontaneous drawings of concepts with some modifications. This made them most recognizable to Charlie, even after a period of time in which he had not needed to refer to those particular pictures or words.

Combining Gestures. During the third week, we began eliciting new gestures and drilling Charlie in their use. We also began to work on providing Charlie with a lexicosyntactic structure for the gesture approach, teaching him ways to combine gestures to express additional concepts. For example, we taught him to convey the color of an object by rubbing the surface of something of that color, after making the gesture for the object itself. This rubbing gesture was intended to be quite distinct from pointing to an object so as not to confuse the listener. We taught Charlie to generalize these simple lexicosyntactic principles in his use of new gestures.

Charlie was also taught to combine gestures with some of the other communication approaches. We taught him to express a variety of concepts related to a single topic through several modalities. For example, we worked on concepts related to shopping for medical supplies. Some of the concepts, such as "'scissors," were best expressed in gestures; others were better expressed using the communication book or by drawing. With this approach, Charlie's master dictionary contained 154 concepts by the end of the fourth week.

Dictionary of Gestures. At this point we began compiling a reference dictionary for family and friends. In addition, we began to reassess his communication needs in light of his impending discharge to his home state. We had asked each member of the family who visited to make a list of subjects they usually discussed with Charlie. With additional discussion we compiled a functional list of subjects and began to direct our training around those topics. At the same time, we organized the dictionary in a similar manner, with a list of pertinent words displayed with the gestures or other techniques by which Charlie conveyed each idea. Unfortunately, we were not able to use pictures or drawings to show the gestures; this meant that some of his closest relatives and friends would not be able to refer to the dictionary because they were unable to read. By way of example, Table 9-3 shows a partial listing for "Fishing" in the dictionary.

During the third week, Charlie's family began to take part in therapy when they were visiting. Most family members were quite adept in understanding common gestures as well as in figuring out new combinations of gestures. With the added help of the dictionary, most family members were able to figure out what Charlie was saying in simple conversations about medical needs, hobbies, recreation, occupations, and so forth. Since the family was able to visit only twice, their training was limited to familiarizing them with the approaches

Table 9–3. Partial Dictionary Listing for the Topic "Fishing"

Fishing	Imitates casting a line
Catfish	Shows size and shape, cat's whiskers
Bass	Writes letter "B," shows size and shape
Salmon	Writes letter "S," shows size and shape
Ocean	Points on map in communication book
Lake	Points on map or draws circle

and teaching them how to solve communication breakdowns. Using the PACE technique again, we taught the family how to narrow down the topic and to verify what was understood as well as how to use the dictionary and to enter new dictionary items.

Discharge Planning. At the end of the fourth week, Charlie was discharged home because his medical needs did not warrant additional hospitalization. Our discharge goals were the following:

1. To provide him with copies of his dictionary and teach him how to teach others to use the booklet.
2. To provide him with a system for emergency phone use at home. He and his family preferred the use of cassette tapes over any system with synthesized speech, such as the Vocaid. We made three tapes to summon an ambulance, a police car, or fire department.
3. To provide him with a yes-no code system for use on the telephone with his family; he used one tap for "yes" and two taps for "no."
4. To provide for his continued treatment by referring him to a Speech Pathologist in his home state, with recommendations that therapy involve the continued assessment of his communication needs and the development of a more flexible communication system that could better meet his needs.

QUESTIONS FOR THE CLINICIAN

Question 1. How did you select the particular gestural approaches you recommended for Charlie? Why didn't you teach him an established sign language, such as American Sign Language, or a standard gestural approach, such as Amer-Ind?

It is important that we recognize the significant differences between the various sign and gestural approaches. Appropriate selection of an approach depends heavily on our understanding of characteristics, such as relative symbolic load, motor complexity, and message flexibility. Only then can we determine whether the specific individuals are able to use the approach and whether it can meet any or all of his or her communication needs (Yorkston and Dowden, 1984).

Symbolic load refers to the extent to which the signs or gestures are arbitrary symbols for the concept they convey. If the relationship is entirely arbitrary or codified, as is the case for much of American Sign Language, both the user and his listeners must be familiar with the "codes." Partners who are unfamiliar with the approach cannot understand the concepts expressed. Some approaches utilize iconic gestures—less symbolic gestures for which there are widely accepted interpretations. For example, American Indian Sign Language (Amer-Ind) utilizes the "thumbs down" gesture to signify "bad." According to Skelly (1979), the gestures are highly intelligible to the untrained viewer because they are signals, not symbols. The third type of gestures, those with the least symbolic load, are those that accompany normal speech. While these "coverbal" gestures carry a great deal of meaning about the speaker and his relationship to his partners, the movements are not symbolic of specific concepts. They are signals in the purest sense.

Message flexibility seems to bear an indirect relationship to the symbolic load. In a system with symbolic gestures, such as American Sign Language, it is possible to communicate any concepts that can be conceived as long as both partners know the symbolic conventions involved. This is not possible with a signal system, however, because the gestures are concrete representations of objects, actions, or persons (Skelly, 1979). Abstract concepts cannot be conveyed except by expanding the system with arbitrary symbols and conventions, which must be learned by the user and all partners.

Motor complexity refers to the type of movements required to produce the gestures. Some signs require complex motor planning in the execution of fine sequential movements. Others involve fewer sequences and grosser movements. Some gestures, for example the coverbal movements, are more or less automatic. Several authors are in the process of assessing the motor control requirements of signing and gestures (Kohl, 1981; Shane and Wilbur, 1980).

Once we are familiar with the characteristics of the approaches under consideration, we must address two critical issues regarding the specific individual. First, we must consider whether a particular gesture or sign approach can meet some or all of the individual's communication needs. Consider the needs that relate to the communication partners. Does the individual need to communicate with anyone who is unfamiliar with the sign or gesture approach? Is it reasonable to expect all partners to learn the approach? Is it possible to use one sign approach for some partners and another with others? In Charlie's case, when he wished to communicate with strangers, an approach with a high symbolic load was not appropriate because the partners could not be trained in their recognition. We chose, instead, to emphasize iconic or referential gestures, such as those found in Amer-Ind. However, many Amer-Ind gestures had to be modified to make them most recognizable to Charlie's family and friends even if the gesture was puzzling to us. For example, Charlie's family understood him immediately when he gestured corn on the cob by pretending to strip the corn from the cob and mix it with a sauce, because that was the way they always ate corn. That gesture was clearly iconic to Charlie's family and friends.

We must also consider the messages or concepts that the individual needs to express. Does he or she need to convey only concrete concepts, or must unique and abstract ideas be expressed? In Charlie's case, he clearly needed to convey abstract ideas, the very concepts that cannot be expressed easily by the universal signals of Amer-Ind. The use of an approach with more symbolic gestures would have permitted him to express the abstract ideas except for two major obstacles: Charlie was not able to learn such an approach in three weeks' time, and his communication partners would not be able to understand the gestures. We were clearly not able to meet Charlie's need to express unlimited and abstract ideas.

The second major consideration, after addressing the issue of communication needs, is the individual's ability to learn a gestural approach. There is a growing body of literature that documents the existence of gestural deficits in nonspeaking adults with language or motor speech impairments (see Chapter 12). The clinician must know whether the nonspeaking individual has any impairment in his or her ability to use symbols or in motor control or motor planning. The existence of such deficits should not preclude the use of gestures altogether, but it should guide decisions about the selection and use of gestures. Charlie showed deficits in motor planning as well as in his ability to learn new symbolic gestures. This necessitated that we avoid the highly symbolic gestural approaches and emphasize the modification of his spontaneous iconic or referential gestures.

ACKNOWLEDGMENTS

Lynn Farrier, the student clinician, contributed significantly to Charlie's program. She was essential to the therapy sessions, but her special contribution was in developing and organizing the gesture dictionary.

REFERENCES

Davis, G. A., and Wilcox, M. J. Incorporating parameters of natural conversation in aphasia treatment: PACE therapy. In R. Chapey (Ed.), *Language intervention strategies in adult aphasia*. Baltimore: Williams & Wilkins, 1981.

Kohl, F. Effects of motoric requirements on the acquisition of manual sign responses by severely handicapped students. *American Journal of Mental Deficiency*, 1981, *85*(4). 396–403.

Shane, H.D., and Wilbur, R.B. Prediction of experience sign potential based on motor control. *Sign Language Studies*, 1980, Winter, pp. 331–48.

Skelly, M. *Amer-Ind gestural code based on universal American Indian hand talk*. New York: Elsevier, 1979.

Yorkston, K.M., and Dowden, P.A. Nonspeech language and communication systems. In A. Holland, (Ed.), *Language disorders in adults: Recent Advances* (pp. 284–312). San Diego: College-Hill Press.

ADDITIONAL READINGS

DeRenzi, E., Motti, F., and Nichelli, P. Imitating gestures: A quantitative approach to ideomotor apraxia. *Archives of Neurology*, 1980, *37*, 6–10.

Griffith, P.L., Robinson, J.H., and Panagos, J.M. Perception of iconicity in American Sign Language by hearing and deaf subjects. *Journal of Speech and Hearing Disorders*, 1981, *46*, 388–397.

Keith, R. L., and Darley, F. L. *Laryngectomee rehabilitation*. San Diego: College-Hill Press, 1979.

Kimura, D. The neurological basis of language qua gesture. In H. Whitaker and H.A. Whitaker (Eds.), *Studies in neurolinguistics* (Vol. 2). New York: Academic Press, 1976.

Oakander, S. *Language board instruction kit*. Fountain Valley, CA: Plavan School, Non Oral Communication Center, 1980.

Skelly, M., Schinsky, L., Smith, R., Donaldson, R., and Griffin, J. American Indian Sign: A gestural system for the speechless. *Archives of Physical Medicine and Rehabilitation*, 1975, *56*, 156–160.

CHAPTER 10

David

Etiology: Head injury
Onset: 17 years of age
Approach: Computer-based auditory scanner and recreational system
Focus: This chapter describes the case of a young man with severe motor impairment and cortical blindness as a result of a head injury. An Apple computer was programmed as an auditory scanning communication system that was controlled by a thumb switch. Inclusion of an Adaptive Peripherals Firmware Card with the Apple system allowed recreational activities.

BACKGROUND

David entered our center at 19 years of age. He had been completely anarthric, with no sound production for speech, for approximately 2 years following extensive head injuries sustained in an automobile accident. In addition to his speechlessness, David was diagnosed as cortically blind, although his parents and teachers reported inconsistent evidence that he could recognize certain people. His severe motor impairment left him dependent upon others to assist him with mobility in his wheelchair, eating, toileting, and dressing. Following the accident, David had lived at home with his parents.

In his parent's home he received regular physical therapy. An attendant assisted the family during the day with David's physical care and exercise program.

At the time he entered our center, David and his family employed two primary communication approaches. Messages were communicated by having the partner verbally scan through the alphabet arrangement presented in Figure 10-1. The partner would say "1, 2, 3, or 4" to offer David the specific row of alphabet letters. David would indicate his choice by adducting his left thumb to squeeze the partner's arm. Next, the communication partner would verbally scan letter by letter and David again would indicate his choice with a thumb squeeze. The partner

1	A	B	C	D	E	F
2	G	H	I	J	K	L
3	M	N	O	P	Q	R
4	S	T	U	V	W	X	Y	Z

Figure 10-1. The alphabet arrangement employed in David's early communication system.

would reformulate the messages on a letter by letter basis. While this communication approach allowed for a wide variety of message types, the communication partners were required to be in close proximity to David; they needed to possess the ability to reformulate the messages that he sent, and they had to take the time necessary to make this communication system successful. Obviously, this was an extremely dependent system, as the partner's had to be in physical contact with David and had to concentrate totally on the communication task. In addition to the dependent verbal scanning communication approach, David learned to signal "yes" and "no" by pointing his left thumb upward for "yes" and downward for "no." He signalled anger, hunger, and dissatisfaction with a full body extension.

EVALUATION

Needs Assessment

David's communication needs were identified during an interview with his mother and his attendant. An attempt was made to have David participate in this interview; however, his slow rate of communication and his inability to analyze his communication needs beyond the present limited his involvement. The results of the needs assessment are presented in Table 10-1. It was mandatory that David communicate in several locations. His communication partners considered it mandatory to be able to communicate with David from across the room, so that they could continue to work on other projects while they interacted with him. Previously they had interrupted their activities to establish physical contact with David, and they found this extremely frustrating and time consuming. The need to communicate with strangers was listed as a desirable rather than a mandatory need,

Table 10-1 David's Communication Needs List

Position	
M	In bed (supine)
M	In wheelchair
M	In bed sitting
Communication Partners	
M	Someone who is across the room or in another room
D	Several people at a time
Locations	
M	In multiple rooms at home
M	In dimly lit rooms
M	In bright sunlight
M	In noisy rooms
Message Needs	
M	Answer yes/no questions

Key: M = Mandatory
D = Desirable but not mandatory

because at the time the needs assessment was completed, David was always accompanied by his attendant or a family member. Upon further reflection it became apparent that if the communication system were successful, David's need to communicate with strangers would probably increase. Because the family desired that David be involved in family activities, the requirements of communicating in noisy rooms, with the rest of the family present, in dimly lit rooms while the family was watching television, and under the bright lights of the patio were considered mandatory communication needs. At the time of the needs assessment, the ability to communicate in the family's van or outside the home was desired but not mandatory. David's mandatory and desired message types included communication, attention getting, answering yes-no questions, requesting assistance using stereotypic phrases, and communicating unique messages in print.

Capability Assessment

Motor Control. David demonstrated a severe and extensive motor impairment. He was unable to walk or stand. His balance and strength for sitting were so limited that he was supported bilaterally by wedges in his wheelchair and by pillows when he sat in bed. His poor head control necessitated a head support mounted on the wheelchair to keep him from lowering his head in neck flexion. His leg movement was limited to the extension of the hips and knees during times of apparent anger or excitement. At the beginning of our intervention, extension of the knee was commonly associated with attempts at voluntary activity of the arm or hands. No voluntary movement of the right hand or arm were observed. There was gross voluntary movement of the left arm with a 12 inch range of movement from his lap to the left side of his body. Independent adduction of the left thumb was observed along with simultaneous flexion of all fingers of the left hand. This movement appeared to be the most reliable of any of his voluntary movements and thus was selected for interface control.

Language.   We found it extremely difficult to test David's language capabilities. Due to his cortical blindness, reading was not tested. Because of the visual and motor requirements of most vocabulary tests, formal evaluation of the vocabulary was impossible. Using the verbal scanning approach described above, we determined that spelling skills were adequate for a communication approach which relied on letter-by-letter message preparation. For example, David demonstrated the ability to spell out his name as well as the names of his family members. He also accurately spelled common requests such as "drink, milk, pop, water, TV, and urinal." He spelled the names of locations such as school, home, bedroom, and bathroom.

Cognition.   We were likewise unable to formally evaluate David's cognitive abilities because of his motoric and visual impairments. Using his dependent verbal scanning communication system, we determined that he was oriented to person and place only. He was inconsistently oriented to time. He was inconsistently aware of events that had occurred earlier in the day of the evaluation. He remembered the names of friends and activities that had occurred prior to the accident. He participated in our attempts to evaluate him for 30 minute periods with regular stimulation from the examiner. We did little to evaluate his learning ability. Evidence suggested a mixed pattern. He had learned to associate the letters grouped by number for the dependent scanning approach described earlier.

Vision.   Several attempts were made to evaluate David's vision. His family, teachers, and friends reported evidence of visual ability. In the classroom, he would respond when he "saw" certain friends enter the room. However, at the time of our initial evaluation, vision specialists reported inconsistent response to their tests. Given limited visual information available, we decided to approach David as though he were completely blind. We felt that we could not depend upon consistent visual function to support a communication approach.

INTERVENTION

Phase One: Development of a Communication System

Introduction of the Thumb Switch. The goal of our first phrase of intervention was to decrease David's dependence on his communication partners by allowing them the freedom to move about while they interacted with him. We retained the basic alphabet scanning approach that was described in the background section of this chapter. However, we provided David with a simple communication aid, which is shown in Figure 10–2. David was able to grasp the interface with his left hand and activate the thumb switch with his left thumb. The switch operates in a momentary rather than a latching fashion. When David depressed the thumb switch, the light or beeper, or both (shown in Figure 10–2), were activated and would remain activated until David released the switch. Using the thumb-switch beeper, the communication partners would verbally scan the alphabet, and David could signal his indications to them across the room or in the car. David successfully incorporated this modification into his day-to-day communication system.

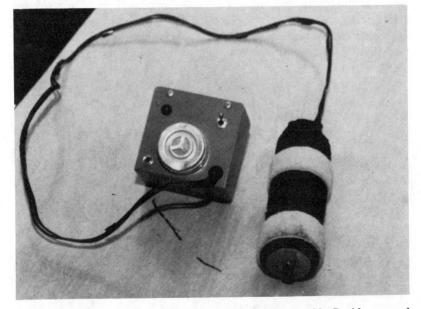

Figure 10–2. A thumb switch – activated light and beeper used by David as an early communication system.

Morse Code Training Trials. The development and use of interface control led to the second aspect of our intervention. This involved an attempt to provide David with an independent communication system which he could control without viewing of the control display or the output display. A Morse code–based communication system was introduced to him. His interface switch was modified, such that the thumb switch was retained while a second switch was positioned beneath the index and middle fingers of his left hand (Fig. 10–3). With a few weeks of training, David demonstrated the ability to activate the thumb switch and the finger switch independently. His interface switch was attached to an A-Tronix Morse code translator, which was used as a training device (see Chapters 3 and 6 for discussion of this training unit). The A-Tronix unit did not provide spoken output, but during the training phase, David's attendant or his mother provided him with spoken output corresponding to the visual display of the A-Tronix system.

Initially, David's Morse code training program focused on the motor control requirements of sending Morse code with a two switch approach. David demonstrated the ability to control each switch independently and to activate alternate switches at an automatic keyer rate, which corresponded to 4 words/minute. Training then focused on learning the codes for the alphabet letters. The alphabet was divided into groups of five letters each. Over the course of 5 months of training by his communication aid and mother, David learned codes for 12 letters. At that point his learning curve plateaued, and his training was discontinued.

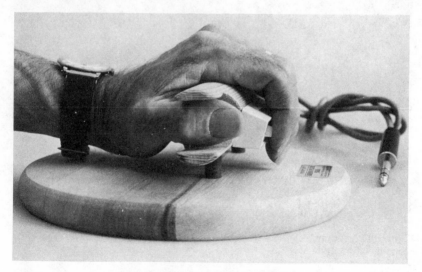

Figure 10–3. David's thumb switch.

Computerization of Auditory Scanning. Another attempt to increase David's communication independence involved the computerization of his initial verbal scanning approach to communication. To accomplish this, an Apple II + computer (with speech synthesis capability via an Echo II Card) was programmed to auditorily scan through options similar to those in his previous dependent approach. The auditory scanning was accompanied by a visual display on the screen (see Fig. 10-4). With his thumb switch, David could interrupt the scan at the number that corresponded to a proper row or the individual letter of choice. Messages were formulated on a letter-by-letter basis. To monitor what he had written and to communicate with persons around him, David could activate a text-to-speech algorithm, by selecting the command "speak" in the command row of the scanning scheme. When a message was completed to his satisfaction, he could print the message by activating the "print" command. Because letter-by-letter message preparation using a scanning approach is extremely slow, a list of frequently used messages was included in the scan menu. The items included in the scan menu were the words, "yes", "no", "maybe", and the following phrases: "I don't know," "Nice to see you," "When will you be back," "Have a nice day," and "Please leave me alone." Subsequently, a message retrieval subroutine was added to the program. A message of choice could be retrieved using a mnemonic code of one or two letters. The messages were selected by David, his attendant, his parents, and the center staff. David selected the message code using the alphabet scan and then indicated the "retrieve"

1	Space	A	B	C	D	E	F		Backspace
2	G	H	I	J	K	L			Backspace
3	M	N	O	P	Q	R			Backspace
4	S	T	U	V	W	X	Y	Z	Backspace

Commands: RETRIEVE   PRINT   SPEAK   CLEAR

Words: YES   NO   MAYBE   MOM   DAD
BOBBY   HELLO   GOODBYE

Numbers: 1   2   3   4   5   6   7   8   9   0

Figure 10-4. David's control display scheme.

command. In response to the "retrieve" command, the entire message was placed in the text which David was formulating. David has used the computer-based auditory scanning system for approximately 2 months. He is able to answer questions; however, he seldom initiates interaction. He does not yet attend to the task long enough to write messages independently.

Phase Two: Development of Computer-Based Recreational Activities

In this phase, we focused on David's recreational activities. His attendant and parents frequently had mentioned David's inability to engage in recreational activity. They considered participation in sustained activity important for the development of cognitive and social skills. The initial phase of this intervention was to provide David and his family with the motor training games developed by Schwejda and McDonald. We were aware that these games were rather elementary for David and were heavily dependent on vision. However, the graphics were very large and we provided a RF Modulator with David's computer system so that the graphics could be displayed on the family's color television set. David's switch was wired into the computer in such a way that it would serve to replace one of the game paddles. Therefore, he was able to operate some of the motor training games with large graphics. During the course of our intervention with David we became increasingly aware of his residual visual abilities when large colored

At the time this case study was being written, other computer games are being prepared for David's use. An Adaptive Peripherals Firmware Card was added to David's computer system. This card provided two important features to support game playing by a severely physically handicapped person. First, the card permits reduction of the speed at which the computer operates and thus slows the rate at which the game is played. With the Firmware Card the rapid cognitive, motor, and visual demands of the games were reduced. Second, software associated with the Firmware Card was be modified so that a variety of games could be played without the joystick type of control, which computer games often require. When joystick control is necessary, the card stops the game and provides a scanning alternative with unlimited time for the individual operating a single switch control. Currently, we are selecting games which David can manage.

QUESTIONS FOR THE CLINICIAN

Question 1. Why were you not able to predict that David would be unable to learn the Morse code at a level necessary for communication system use?

At the time of this intervention, we knew very little about predicting the potential of anyone to learn Morse code. We chose to take a risk because we reasoned that if we were successful in teaching Morse code, David would have a system with the potential to be more rapid than the auditory scanning system. We did not succeed in our training. Fortunately, we had an inexpensive Morse code translation device available to use during the trial, so we did not expend equipment money unnecessarily. Results from the Alternative Communication System project (Wilson, 1981) completed at the University of Washington, Seattle, demonstrated that children with cerebral palsy who had attained third grade spelling skills were able to learn Morse code without exception. As professionals, we have little useful information in predicting the potential of a client to learn the skills associated with communication system control. This remains a very important area of clinical research.

Question 2. How was the specialized computer software developed for David?

Development of individualized software on a clinical rather than a research basis is an important concern in this field. On David's behalf, we utilized clinical and research staff to develop the software. The use of research staff was justified, as this was a new approach to communication augmentation that was initially described in an article published by Beukelman, Traynor, Poblette, and Warren (1984). As computers become more frequently employed in this field, the need for clinical programmers will become mandatory. An alternative may be private companies that write and modify software to meet the needs of the individual client. Currently, the Trace Software Directory provides a listing of communication augmentation software. Occasionally, standard software meets a nonspeaking individual's needs. However, individualization is often necessary.

Question 3. What are the differences between operating auditory and visual scan?

In our opinion, operating audio scan is more difficult than visual scan. In the visual scan mode, the user can view the entire array, while in audio scan, the users must memorize the array if they are going to present a letter or command. When nonimpaired individuals operated audio scan, we found that they did not respond as quickly to the audio as to the visual presentation of the letter. Therefore, the scan rate must be slower for audio than visual scan. Ignoring auditory distractions while using audio scan is more difficult than ignoring visual distractions while operating visual scan. Figure 10–4 show that we retained the alphabetical order arrangement for the auditory scan program. An arrangement in which the letters were ordered by frequency of occurrence makes it much more difficult to anticipate letter presentation.

Question 4. For what other type of application would the audioscan approach be used?

We believe that audioscan will be useful in cases in which the nonspeaking individual has difficulty seeing a visual control display. David was unable to use the display because of cortical blindness. Another of our clients, Terry, is using audioscan because his motor control problems are so severe that he cannot maintain sustained visual contact with a visual control display. We evaluated Terry for the first time when he was 13 years old. He has very severe spastic cerebral palsy with a very active right asymmetric tonic neck reflex (ATNR), which rotates his head to the extreme right. During the reflex, he is unable to maintain visual contact with a display positioned before him. Terry used tongue clicks and occasionally produced speech which could be understood by his parents. Involuntary inspiratory stridor was frequently present, especially during times of excitement. His communication system consisted of "twenty questions," with one tongue-click for "no," two clicks for "yes," and three clicks for "maybe" and "I don't know." He also spontaneously spelled some words using the dependent verbal scan similar to that described for David, in which the listener spoke the alphabet in segments and Terry clicked his tongue to indicate his choice of row and letter. Terry also used a communication board in a dependent scanning mode with persons from school; however, this approach was not used at home.

Terry was referred to our center by personnel from his school district. Despite years of effort to develop Terry's linguistic skills and the communication approaches described above, they were experiencing difficulty increasing his communicative independence because of the difficulty in developing an interface. Terry demonstrated no voluntary control over his arms, legs, or head rotation. With the help of a volunteer, the school personnel had developed a prototype "tongue switch" (Littleman and Costigan, 1983). When Terry protruded his tongue to contact a plate positioned anterior to his lips, he closed an electrical circuit. At the time of referral, Terry was demonstrating inconsistent use of the tongue switch during motor training exercises but was not controlling an independent communication system. His inability to maintain visual contact with a control screen was proving to be a barrier in his program.

When Terry came for an evaluation, we had just finished designing David's system. In fact the system had not yet been delivered. We involved Terry in a trial with the audioscan program. Terry

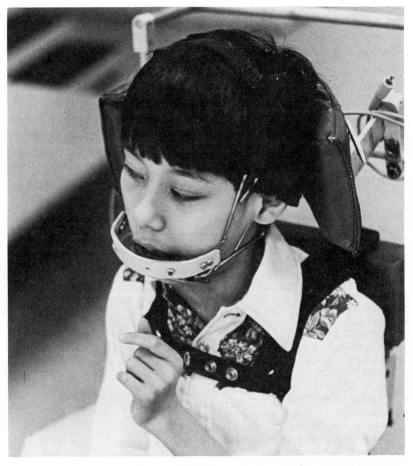

Figure 10-5. Terry's tongue switch.

demonstrated his understanding of the approach in just a few minutes. His use of the tongue switch was too inconsistent to control the system in a completely independent manner, so we controlled the system for him as he clicked his tongue to signal switch closures. Within a half an hour, Terry was spelling words using this approach.

To increase the efficiency of Terry's tongue switch control, we reconfigured the switch slightly (Fig. 10-5). The touch plate was enlarged in comparison to the prototype. The bar on which the touch plate was mounted was made adjustable, so that the plate could be more effectively positioned. With the modified switch, we gave Terry a second trial with the audioscan system. This time he used the system independently. When possible he viewed the computer monitor and worked in a visual scan mode; however, during times when his head rotated far to the right, he used the system in the audioscan mode.

During the early months of Terry's use of the system, he practiced with it at school, using equipment belonging to the school district. Before delivering his software, we programmed a message retrieval capability. Terry, his parents, and school personnel suggested messages that were to be retrieved. A list of these messages along with their retrieval codes is given in Table 10-2. At the time this chapter was written, Terry had used the system for approximately 3 months. School personnel report that he began to use the message retrieval functions immediately. The time savings apparently appealed to him. The overall slowness of message preparation (letter by letter spelling) of the system is very apparent.

Table 10-2. Message Units and Their Retrieval Codes Programmed for Terry's Audio Scan System

Messages	Retrieval Codes	Program Line
Feelings		
I want to quit	WQ	2047
I'm mad	IM	2025
I like	IL	2026
I love you	LY	2027
I'm happy	IH	2028
I'm upset	AU	2029
I want to	IW	2030
I don't want to	DW	2031
Don't bug me	DB	2032
Be like a banana and split	LB	2033
Narrative		
I went out to dinner	WD	2034
We had company at our house	HC	2035
My dad is out-of-town	OT	2036
We make juggling equipment	JE	2037
I watched TV	TV	2038
I went shopping	WS	2039
I went to a baseball game	BG	2040
Physical Needs		
I feel sick	FS	2041
I'm tired	IT	2042
I need to go to the bathroom	BR	2043
I want to get out of my wheelchair	OC	2044
I want to get into my wheelchair	IC	2045
I'm uncomfortable in my chair	UC	2046
Please move my chair	MC	2048
I want to lie down	LD	2053
I'm cold	AC	2054
I'm hot	AH	2055
School Needs		
My favorite class is	FC	2052
When is lunch?	WL	2050
What are we going to eat?	WE	2051
I didn't do it	DD	2049

Table 10–2 (continued)

Interaction

Hello, how are you doing?	HI	2006
My name is Terry	NA	2001
Do you understand?	UN	2002
What is your name?	WY	2003
I'll start over	ST	2004
I need help	HE	2005
Please repeat what you heard, after I speak	RE	2007
That's all	TA	2008
The subject is	SU	2009
Would you like to wait for the answer or come back in a minute?	CB	2010
I don't know	DK	2011
I don't want to answer	DW	2011
I use this system to talk	IU	2013
I can hear just fine. Speak naturally to me, please	IH	2014
What did you say?	WH	2015
Please wait	PW	2016
I can't remember	CR	2017
Ask me yes/no questions	YN	2018
Tell me more	TM	2019
What do you think?	WT	2020
Let's talk about baseball	TB	2056
I don't understand	DU	2022
See you later	SY	2023
Please give me	GM	2024
What's new?	WM	2020

We are working to develop a device that will transduce the tongue click into a switch closure and at the same time ignore environmental noise and Terry's inspiratory stridor. However, even if we are successful, this efficient switch probably will not change the overall message preparation speed in an important way. Right now we are attempting to increase Terry's communication interaction speed by increasing the number of messages he can retrieve. The reader is referred to several articles in the *Additional Readings* section that deal with message retrieval and communication speed. Certainly our continuing efforts on Terry's behalf will be to enhance the speed of message preparation, an issue that is going to occupy the communication augmentation field for years to come.

ACKNOWLEDGMENTS

We would like to acknowledge the help of several individuals for their contributions to this case study. Miguel Poblette provided initial software suggestions. Gregg Tuai provided the final version of the software. Charles Traynor provided frequent consultation regarding computer applications. Russ Paul, Marvin Soderquist, and Bruce Terami provided technical, electrical, and mechanical solutions. We wish to thank David and his parents for their extensive patience which permitted us to fail on occasion as we attempted to develop this communication system. Terry's tongue switch was developed by the staff from the Edmonds, Washington, School District together with their volunteers, Paul Schwejda and Steve Date. Their support of David through the years has been substantial.

REFERENCES

Beukelman, D. R., Traynor, C.D., Poblette, M., and Warren, G. Microcomputer based communication augmentation systems for two nonspeaking physically handicapped persons with severe visual impairment. *Archives of Physical Medicine and Rehabilitation*, 1984, *65*, 89–91.

Littleman, V. A., and Costigan, C.L. One-function tongue interface for a child with severe cerebral palsy, *Proceedings of the 6th Annual Conference of the Rehabilitation Engineering Society of North America*, 1983, *6*, 248.

Wilson, W. An alternative communication system for the severely physically handicapped. Grant # 6007804512 Handicapped Media Services and Captioned Films Program, Washington, DC: Department of Education, 1981.

ADDITIONAL READINGS

Cote-Baldwin, C. Use of the Apple II microcomputer with physically handicapped children. Computers and the handicapped. Ottawa: Research Council of Canada, 1982, pp. 107–114.

Levin, H. S., Benton, A. L., and Rossman, R. G. *Neurobehavioral consequences of closed head injury*. New York: Oxford University Press, 1982.

Schwejda, P., and Vanderheiden, G. Adaptive Firmware Card for the Apple II. *Byte*, 1982, *7*, 276–317.

CHAPTER 11

Jeff

Etiology: Cerebral palsy
Onset: Congenital
Approach: Dependent auditory scanning approach; ScanWRITER
Focus: This chapter illustrates the case of a 26 year old community college student with severe athetoid cerebral palsy. Overflow movements prevented him from using head or eye-gaze movements to access a communication augmentation system. The system selected for him was a footswitch–controlled ScanWRITER. We discuss issues of computer-keyboard emulation and maximizing message preparation rates in scanning systems.

BACKGROUND

In 1980, Jeff came to the Engineering Applications Program located at the University of Washington Hospital with considerable information about his own abilities and the potential of electronics to meet his educational and communication needs. Through the years he had anticipated that someday he might be able to use a Morse code–based approach as an alternative means of communication and had expended the effort to learn the code.

Because of Jeff's severe physical involvement, a suitable interface had not been developed for him. He had extremely severe athetoid cerebral palsy. He sat in an individualized seat mounted to a wheelchair frame. Due to extensive movement patterns during rest and voluntary activity, his chair was equipped with an electric fan to cool him. He used the fan when electrical power was available. His hands were restrained, as were his legs. Jeff made no voluntary sound with the exception of a tongue click. He was completely dependent in terms of walking, feeding, and toileting.

At the time Jeff came to the Engineering Application Program, he was communicating using a partner-dependent auditory scanning system, similar to that employed by David and described in Chapter 10. His communication partner would scan the alphabet and Jeff would

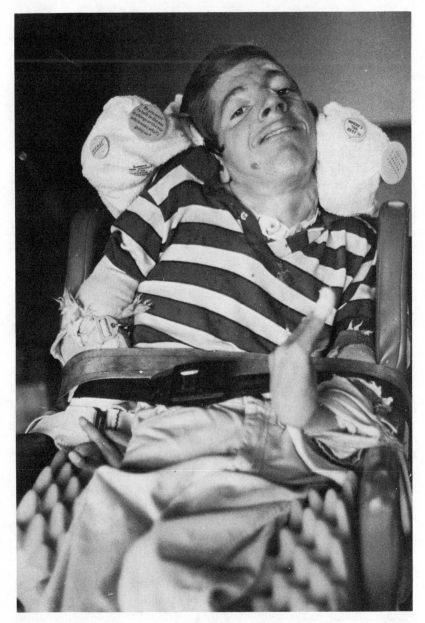

Figure 11-1. Jeff seated in his wheelchair. Note his "communication button" (on the far right) containing the alphabet arrangement he uses for auditory scanning.

use eye-gaze to signal "yes." He signaled "no" with a gross head
rotation and clicked his tongue to signal that he wished to communicate.
Figure 11–1 shows Jeff in his wheelchair. Note the button attached
to the headrest on the far right of the photo (on Jeff's left) displays
the alphabet arrangement of Jeff's auditory scanning system.
Communication partners refer to the button to refresh their memory
about the scanning arrangement. Only those individuals very familiar
and committed to Jeff would attempt to communicate with him.
Therefore, he had little opportunity to communicate with strangers or
with the other residents in the cerebral palsy residential center where
he lived. He also communicated with a Tufts Interactive Communicator
(TIC), which is a row-column scanning communication system with no
message retrieval, a ticker tape printout, and a marquee-type screen.
The system is not portable and is powered with 110 volt wall power.
He accessed the TIC with a foot switch designed by a friend (Fig. 11–2).
The switch was mounted on his right footrest. Jeff activated the switch
by extending his foot forward. As is shown in Figure 11–2, his foot
is strapped to the switch.

The goal of the Engineering Application Program staff was to select
an interface for Jeff so that he could access a Morse code–based
communication system. Under the direction of Gerald Warren, director
of the program at the time, a research project was begun to develop

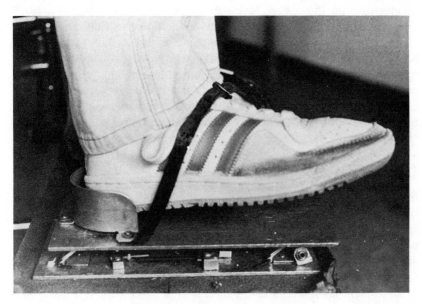

Figure 11–2. Jeff's footswitch.

an eye-gaze switch. A crude prototype was developed by the program, and when it was held in position, Jeff demonstrated the ability to activate the switch by gazing laterally and upward. A more complete prototype was developed by Zygo Industries (Tigard, OR). Although Jeff could activate the switch through eye gaze, this interface was never used to access a communication system, for several reasons. First, the combination of Jeff's overflow movements and the contact pressure between the back and sides of his headrest and the glasses frames on which the eye-gaze sensors were mounted constantly moved the frames out of position. Consequently, the rapid movements required to send Morse code could not be maintained. Second, the involvement of the eyes in the switch control precluded the use of visual contact with the control display of a scanning communication system. At the conclusion of the unsuccessful effort to provide an eye-gaze interface for Jeff, he was referred to our center for further attempts to provide him with an independent communication system.

EVALUATION

Needs Assessment

The communication needs assessment was completed by Jeff, his attendant, and the speech-language pathologist from the residential center (Table 11–1). A review of this table indicates that Jeff needed to produce unique messages in several formats, including papers for school. He wished to communicate with a number of different partners and in a number of environments. Finally, his unique needs included access to a computer and some special considerations related to system mounting. He also indicated that in the future he wished to reside in an independent living center, so the communication system would have to meet his needs there.

Capability Assessment

Motor Control. As was mentioned previously, Jeff was severely limited physically, with no voluntary movement of the hands and arms. He demonstrated slight rotary movement of the head when it was positioned against the headrest. The level of control was not adequate for direct selection access because of overflow movements and lack of fine control. To suppress overflow movements, his hands and arms were secured with straps, and his head was stabilized against a headrest. His left leg was also secured. There was some consistent extension of

Table 11-1. Listing of Jeff's Mandatory Communication Needs

Message Types
>Unique messages
>Stereotyped messages for self-care and health care, and
>>conversational management
>Memos to staff and residents
>Letters
>Papers for school

Communication Partners
>Reading and nonreading residents at the
>>residential center
>Staff at the center
>Students and faculty at college
>Strangers
>Family

Environment
>Residential Center
>College
>Field trips and outings
>Home

Other needs
>Access to a computer for educational and prevocational activities
>Size and positioning of communication equipment to permit frequent
>>care and feeding activities by staff

the right leg at the knee and hip. Jeff exhibited moderately severe scoliosis.

Vision. Our evaluation revealed that Jeff could read and recognize letters on the control displays as small as three eighths inch. He was able to read the print from a conventional typewriter. He could direct his eye gaze voluntarily and fix his eyes on a target even when his head was moving about as a result of overflow activity.

Language. The language assessment was completed primarily by the speech-language pathologist from Jeff's residential center. His performance on the Peabody Picture Vocabulary Test (Dunn, 1965) placed him at the ceiling of the test (18.5 year level. His Wide Range Achievement Test (Jastak and Jastak, 1965) spontaneous spelling score placed him at the 9.2 grade level. On the Gates-MacGinitie Reading Test (Gates and MacGinitie, 1965, 1969), he scored at the 10.6 grade level. Since Jeff demonstrated the language ability to manage a spelling-based communication system, and since he was already spelling for most of his communication, we did no further assessment of linguistic or cognitive skills.

INTERVENTION

System Selection

Morse Code.   With the foot switch available to us, we evaluated Jeff again with the idea of deciding between a Morse code–based communication system and a row-column scanning system. While Jeff could occasionally make the appropriate movements for single switch Morse code control at a very slow rate, the physical effort required for such an application appeared to be excessive for Jeff. After a few minutes of Morse code practice he was sweating profusely. Jeff had long preferred to use a Morse code–based system and had taken the time at a much younger age to learn Morse code, hoping some day to make use of it for communication. However, for the time being, we abandoned Morse code–based options.

Scanning.   Jeff demonstrated single switch control adequate to access a row-column scanning communication system. We selected a new product, the ScanWRITER, manufactured by Zygo Industries, Inc. (Fig. 11–3). The ScanWRITER was selected for several reasons. This system provides scanning control for a single switch user. It allows letter-by-letter spelling for unique messages, but also allows some message retrieval for self-care and health care needs as well as conversational management. The ScanWRITER also serves as a keyboard emulator for the Apple II+ and IIe computers. Messages can be prepared on a paper strip wide enough to contain a 20 character line; messages can also be spoken with a text-to-speech algorithm. This device would allow Jeff to communicate through speech to nonreading residents as well as to staff members and strangers in conversational situations. The printed option would allow preparation of messages, letters, and assignments. The ScanWRITER does not permit 8 by 11 inch formatting of type. However, when Jeff has computer access, he will write with a word processing program and a conventional printer. A final reason for selecting the ScanWRITER was its relatively small size. Because Jeff needs such extensive care, the small size of the ScanWRITER allows the staff, family members, and attendants easy access to him.

Future Directions.   We continue to attempt to improve the efficiency of Jeff's access to the ScanWRITER. Currently, we are developing a new foot switch for him. The design goal is to provide a switch that will allow greater range of movement, so that his foot does not have to be so carefully positioned to activate the switch. Perhaps the most potentially promising work takes a quite different direction and is being attempted by a graduate student of engineering. The goal of this work is to develop a circuit that will transduce Jeff's tongue clicks into a switch closure while ignoring the environmental sounds around him. This project was also referred to in Chapter 10.

QUESTIONS FOR THE CLINICIAN

Question 1. What are the unique problems experienced by an individual who attempts to use a communication augmentation system as a keyboard emulator?

There are several benefits as well as several problems. The use of the same interface for communication as for computer control is a great benefit for the individual who is severely disabled. The "best" motor

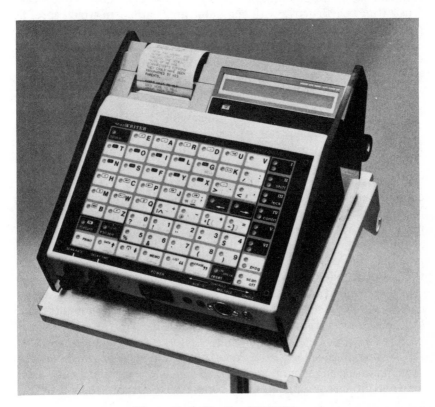

Figure 11-3. The ScanWRITER.

control pattern can be used for both functions. Some functions of the communication augmentation system can be used to enhance the efficiency of computer control. For example, commonly used terms, such as RUN, PRINT, GOTO, and LIST, can be retrieved as messages from the memory of the communication augmentation system and do not need to be spelled in their entirety each time they are used.

On the negative side, when the communication augmentation system is used as a keyboard emulator, its function as a communication device is limited or eliminated. For example, if the user is working on the computer and someone comes in to talk, the communication system may not be available for conversational interactions. This is probably an even larger problem in vocational settings, as communication with fellow employees may be necessary while the user is working on a computer. Another problem may arise when the communication augmentation system requires visual contact with a control screen. As users are working with a computer, they are required to shift back and forth between the computer monitor and the control display of the communication augmentation system. At times users find this frustrating, particularly with computer applications in which careful control of cursor function is required.

Question 2.   What are the unique requirements of a communication augmentation system that is used by a college student in a departmentalized educational setting?

Obviously, there is the need for a portable, reliable communication system. When a student travels from class to class in a wheelchair, often there is minimal time to make the transition, let alone set up an elaborate communication system. It is essential that college students take notes in class. The communication augmentation system should support this activity. However, it should be acknowledged that most communication augmentation system users cannot achieve the message preparation rate to be good note takers. The brief notes taken by the system user must always be supplemented with tape recordings of the lectures, with copies of notes taken by nondisabled students, or with the aid of an educational attendant.

The preparation of written assignments requires special consideration. Usually the printed output of the communication augmentation system does not conform to the 8 x 11 inch format required in college courses. For shorter papers, the student should ask for permission to submit brief reports on the format produced by the communication augmentation system. For longer assignments, the user may need to hire a typist or use a computer to prepare reports in the appropriate format.

Completion of examinations may also require special accommodations for the severely physically disabled individual. Usually, the communication augmentation system user will require additional time to complete examinations. Some test formats are particularly difficult, such as fill-in-the-blank and computer scored answer sheets.

Participation in class is also a concern. Frequently, the nonspeaking individual is excluded from class discussion. At other times, participation is limited to answering yes-no questions. When a longer question is asked, the communication augmentation system user may be required to compose a response while the remainder of the class is continuing the discussion, thus eliminating the user from the benefit of the ensuing discussion or lecture. We often suggest that faculty involve the nonspeaking individuals in a discussion by asking a question at the end of a class period; their answers can be presented at the beginning of the discussion period of the next class period, allowing the nonspeaking individual to prepare the answer outside class time.

Question 3. What approaches may be taken to increase message preparation rates?

Of course, the first approach to maximizing the message preparation rate of a nonspeaking individual is to ensure that the user can reliably control the device and that physical, linguistic, or cognitive limitations prevent the user from operating a more efficient system. Some message preparation rate enhancement techniques appear to impact positively on users of direct selection as well as scanning and encoding systems. Many communication systems allow the user to select complete words and phrases in a message retrieval mode. If words and phrases that are used frequently by the individual can be identified and stored in the device, message preparation rates will be increased accordingly. To investigate the redundancy of word and phrase use, Beukelman and Yorkston (1982) collected the communication samples produced by five adult Canon Communicator users. The preliminary results indicated that a large proportion of the total vocabulary sample consisted of a relatively small list of frequently occurring words. Specifically, the 500 most frequently used words represented 85% of the sample. The number of "slots" needed to communicate a large proportion of the total message is well within the memory and storage capabilities of current technology.

Another issue explored with this data base is "Do messages with similiar communicative intents occur frequently enough so that programming general statements of intent will increase message preparation efficiency?" In order to answer this question, we separated the messages produced by four nonspeaking adults in categories according to the intent of the message. The resulting data are displayed in Table 11-2. A review of this table reveals that there is relatively little redundancy of message intents. For example, 97% of the messages that were categorized as "provision of information" were judged to be unique from other messages. Although the degree of message uniqueness no doubt depends on a variety of factors, including the communication task and environment, along with the linguistic and cognitive capabilites of the individual, uniqueness of messages appears to be a characteristic communication by language-intact adults. Subsequent clinical work with a variety of users of communication augmentation systems with message retrieval has revealed that individuals with spontaneous spelling ability adequate to produce all messages of choice often prefer not to use the message retrieval mode, but prefer to spell all messages in their entirety. When questioned about this preference, they frequently point out that they prefer to retain the message flexibility offered in letter-by-letter spelling. On the other hand, communication augmentation system users with more limited spelling abilities often make prompt and effective use of message retrieval.

Another approach to enhancement of message preparation rates is computer-based prediction of message completion. A language prediction system developed by Paul Schwejda is operating in a Morse code–based alternative communication system (Wilson, 1981). As the first letter of a word is selected, the user is offered on a control display the most probable completion of the word. If the "guess" is correct,

Table 11-2. Number and percentages of Total and Unique Messages Produced by Four Adults Communication Augmentation System Users

	Number of Messages	Percentage of Total Messages	Number of Unique Messages	Percentage of Unique Messages
Provide information	2114	62	2060	97
Request information	669	20	596	89
Request physical assistance	223	7	166	74
Request other assistance	180	6	164	91
Emotional expression	148	5	112	76
Social amenities	39	1	25	64

From Beukelman, D., and Yorkston, K. Communication interaction of adult communication augmentation system use. *Topics in Language Disorders*, 1982, *2*(2), 39–54. Used with permission.

the user selects a space and the completed word is accepted. If the "guess" is incorrect, the user selects the second letter of the desired word and with this additional information the computer "guesses" again. The process continues until the computer guesses correctly or until the word is spelled correctly letter by letter. Linguistic information, such as verb tense, number, and word order, is incorporated into the program to enhance the prediction ability. Preliminary results reveal that approximately 40% of the letters sent in message preparation are generated by the predictive program, with 60% of the letters spelled by the user (Marriner, personal communication). The use of a linguistic prediction program works especially well with a Morse code–based communication augmentation system. Because the users have memorized the code, they do not have to retain visual contact with the control display, as do users of scanning systems and most users of direct selection systems. Therefore, users of the Morse code system can retain visual contact with the screen which displays linguistic predictions, accepting and rejecting options very rapidly. The users of scanning and direct selection systems must visually shift from the control display to the linguistic prediction display.

Message preparation rate can also be enhanced by systems in which the retrieval units are larger than individual sounds or letters. Goodenough-Trepagnier and Prather (1981) have suggested an approach called SPEEC (Sequences of Phonemes for Efficient English Communication). This system contains frequently occurring sequences of sounds, which can be combined by the user to form a message. WRITE is a similar system by the same authors, which contains frequently occurring sequences of letters and can be used for writing. These systems have the advantage of increasing message preparation rates while allowing the user to produce an unrestricted number of unique messages. Still another approach to enhancement of message preparation rates is to optimize entry locations. Goodenough-Trepagnier and Rosen (1981) suggested a computer-based model for deriving the "best key set" for a nonspeaking individual once motor and linguistic capabilities have been assessed.

For the individual using a scanning-type communication augmentation system, the arrangement of letters, numbers, and word(s) on the control display has an important influence on message preparation rate. Beukelman and Poblette (1981) reported a computer simulation of row-column scanning systems in which the relative efficiencies of selected letter and vocabulary arrangements were compared. The interactions among frequency of word and letter occurrence, word length, and scan time for specific control display arrangements are complex. A microcomputer was programmed to simulate the operation of a row-column scanner, and specific display arrangements were programmed into the computer model. The computer program calculated the time required to communicate a standard sample using various display arrangements. Results indicate that letters arranged in the left upper area of the display according to frequency of occurrence are associated with a communication rate that is 13% faster than an A to Z arrangement in the upper left hand corner. Addition of entire words permits communication that is faster than letter-by-letter spelling only if words are selected and entered in the scan display on the basis of frequency of occurrence, word length, and competitive placement. The combination of letters arranged according to frequency of occurrence and selected words on the control display as described previously resulted in a 26% reduction in time for message preparation compared with an A to Z alphabet arrangement only. It should be noted that some users are unable to accurately use or tolerate an alphabetical arrangement according to frequency of occurrence and must use the more familiar A through Z arrangement.

The area of enhancing message preparation rate is a critical one in the field of communication augmentation. Computer-based approaches offer intriguing possibilities. However, we have much to learn about how to increase the efficiency of system use. At a minimum, we need to explore human factors, such as motor control, visual abilities, linguistic skills, and distraction-frustration levels, which may interact with the approaches described above.

ACKNOWLEDGMENTS

We would like to acknowledge the efforts of the staff at Zygo Industries, Inc., for their cooperation throughout this application. Kathy Smith, speech-language pathologist at Jeff's residential center, was also a consistent and important contributor to this effort. Advice from Marvin Soderquist, Russ Paul, and Gerry Warren of the Engineering Applications Program of University of Washington Hospital was appreciated. Dean Tougas designed and built Jeff's foot switch.

REFERENCES

Beukelman, D. R., and Poblette, M. Maximizing communication rates of row-column scanning communication augmentation systems. Paper presented at the American Speech-Language-Hearing Association Convention, Los Angeles, 1981.

Beukelman, D., and Yorkston, K. Communication interaction of adult communication augmentation system use. *Topics in Language Disorders*, 1982, *2*(2), 39–54.

Dunn, L. M. *Expanded manual for the Peabody Picture Vocabulary Test*. Circle Pines, MN: American Guidance Service, 1965.

Gates, A. I., and MacGinitie, W. H. *Gates-MacGinitie Reading Test.* New York: Teacher's College Press, Columbia University, 1965, 1969.

Goodenough-Trepagnier, C., and Prather, P. Communication systems for the nonvocal based on frequent phoneme sequences. *Journal of Speech and Hearing Disorders,* 1981, *24,* 322–329.

Goodenough-Trepagnier, C., and Rosen, M. J. Model for a computer-based procedure to prescribe optimal "keyboards." Presented at the 4th Annual Conference on Rehabilitation Engineering, Washington, DC, 1981.

Jastak, J. F., and Jastak, S.R. *The Wide Range Achievement Test manual.* Wilmington, DE: Guidance Associates, 1965.

Wilson, W. An alternative communication system for the severely physically handicapped. Grant #6007804512 Handicapped Media Services and Captioned Films Program, Department of Education, 1981.

ADDITIONAL READING

Vanderheiden, G. C. Technology needs of individuals with communication impairments. *Seminars in Speech and Language,* 1984, *5*(1), 59–67.

CHAPTER 12

Dallas

Etiology: Left cerebrovascular accident (CVA)
Onset: 47 years old
Approach: Communication books, gestures; Handivoice 130
Focus: This chapter illustrates the case of an interior designer who suffered a left CVA, which resulted in both language deficits and apraxia of speech. During the course of his rehabilitation, he used a number of approaches to augmentation communication, including communication books and gestures. His return to work necessitated a portable, speech synthesis system with a unique vocabulary suited to his design work.

BACKGROUND

A speech-language pathologist met Dallas in the intensive care unit (ICU) of a neighboring hospital. Dallas had arrived there on an emergency basis with progressive weakness of his right arm and leg and difficulty speaking. The speech-language pathologist was consulted because the ICU staff was having difficulty communicating with Dallas and he was becoming increasingly frustrated. Initial screening revealed that Dallas did not speak understandably, and he appeared to comprehend approximately 50% of yes/no questions. Nuclear medicine studies revealed no blood flow in the left middle cerebral and left anterior cerebral arteries. His medical diagnosis was a left cerebral vascular accident (CVA). After Dallas's condition was stabilized medically, he was transferred to the rehabilitation service of the hospital in which our Center was located.

Prior to his hospitalization, Dallas had enjoyed excellent health, with only a slight blood pressure problem which appeared to be controlled without medication. Dallas was 47 years old and owned and managed a successful interior design firm. He taught interior design and served as department chairperson in a local art institute. He was married and the father of three teenaged children, who lived at home.

INITIAL EVALUATION

Communication Needs Assessment

A preliminary needs assessment was completed by Dallas's wife, his primary nurse, and a speech-language pathologist. Obviously, his communication needs were quite different during his rehabilitation program than they would be following his discharge. His needs were quite typical of those for individuals involved in an active rehabilitation program. In addition, the sudden nature of his stroke necessitated extensive communication with employees and clients about business matters. It was decided that contact with clients would not be permitted and that business-related communication would be managed through one employee rather than a group of employees.

Capability Assessment

Language. Upon beginning the rehabilitation program, a Porch Index of Communicative Abilities (PICA) (Porch, 1967) was administered. The PICA is a standardized test used with aphasic patients to give an indication of the severity of language deficits. Dallas's performance on this test in 18 different language tasks could be compared with that of a large sample of individuals with left hemisphere damage. His overall performance placed him at the 22nd percentile. This means that 22% of individuals with left hemisphere damage tested in the normalization sample performed more poorly than he did, and 78% performed better. The PICA, which was administered at 1 month following onset, indicated severely impaired language performance across all modalities:

> Overall average = 22nd percentile
> Gestural average = 20th percentile
> Verbal average = 10th percentile
> Graphic average = 39th percentile

The PICA contains eighteen 10-item subtests measuring communicative behaviors in the verbal, gestural, and graphic modalities. Dallas was able to perform none of the verbal tasks, even the simplest tasks, which require that he imitate single words. We informally tested speech-related oral movements and found that he was able to protrude his tongue only with great difficulty. Although he appeared to understand the task, he was unable to move his tongue from side to side. He was unable to elicit phonation voluntarily but produced a voice when coughing. No spontaneous or imitative verbalizations were noted during the first month following the CVA. Despite aphasia and severe apraxia of speech, which is characterized by severe impairments on speech-related tasks, Dallas performed reflexive or automatic chewing and swallowing activities adequately.

On tasks that required him to listen and follow verbal instructions, deficits were also evident, but they were not as severe as the verbal deficits. For example, two of the auditory comprehension subtests of the PICA required that Dallas listen to the name of an object or listen to a description of the function of the object and then point to the appropriate object in a field of ten. Dallas correctly identified 6 of 10 objects on this task. Deficits were also noted on reading tasks. When asked to match written phrases containing the name of an object to that object, Dallas correctly matched only 1 of 10 items. Gestural output was assessed on the PICA with a task in which Dallas was asked to demonstrate the function of common objects, such as a comb or a table knife. He produced only two recognizable gestures. Results of our initial evaluation led to the diagnosis of moderately severe aphasia accompanied by severe apraxia of speech.

Dallas's interactions with family and staff consisted primarily of responses to yes-no questions. However, communication breakdowns were very common, as his responses to yes-no questions was inconsistently accurate. Breakdowns often went unresolved if family or staff could not lead him successfully though a series of yes-no questions. In order to successfully resolve breakdowns with yes-no questions, the responder must be quite accurate in the response that is provided. A single "wrong" answer can mislead the communication partners and cause them to pursue a line of questioning that will lead in the wrong direction.

Cognitive. Attempts were made to have Dallas complete the performance subtests of the Wechsler Adult Intelligence Scale (WAIS) (Wechsler, 1955) within the first month following the CVA. No attempts were made to have him perform any of the verbal tasks at that time because of his aphasia. With the omission of the "digit-symbol" subtest, his prorated performance IQ was 69, with extreme inter-test scatter. This inter-test scatter gives us the indication that his premorbid performance on these tasks would have been superior, but that significant deficits had occurred as the results of the CVA. His scaled scores on the block design, picture arrangement, and object assembly tasks ranged from 0 to 4 (with 10 being an average adult performance) which appeared to reflect a spatial-perceptual impairment. On Raven's Progressive Matrices Test (Raven, 1960), Dallas achieved a raw score of 22, which is in the lower one fifth of adult performance. All of the cognitive testing behaviors reflected "neurologic confusion" during this initial evaluation.

Portions of the neuropsychological assessment were readministered 2½ months following onset. Results revealed a "dramatic improvement in motor control and spatial-perceptual capabilities." Dallas's performance on Raven's Progressive Matrices test had improved 30 percentile points, from the 20th to the 50th percentile. Scores on the performance subtests of the WAIS had also improved to within the normal range of performance on those subtests that did not require speech.

Motor.   Dallas demonstrated the classic hemiplegia pattern associated with a severe left CVA. He had no functional movement of his right hand or arm. In time, he was able to walk with a brace on his right leg. No impairment of movement with his left hand or leg was observed. By the end of his rehabilitation program, Dallas was able to walk for short distances with the right leg brace and a cane in his left hand. For longer distances or difficult terrain, he used a manual wheelchair, which he propelled with his left foot and hand.

Vision.   Dallas wore reading glasses at the time of his CVA. No change of prescription was required after the stroke. He demonstrated no field cuts or additional acuity problems.

INTERVENTION

Phase I. The First Year

Communication Books.   The first year following onset of aphasia is a time when the majority of changes related to spontaneous recovery occur. In the most general sense, the goal of intervention during the first year is to maximize the recovery of language function. Typically this takes the form of a program of general language retraining accompanied by frequent reassessment of changing performance on speaking, listening, reading, and writing tasks.

Although our initial testing had indicated deficits in all of the language modalities, we initially focused on training auditory comprehension skills. We began training listening tasks rather than speech or gestural output tasks for a number of reasons. First, our initial testing showed that Dallas achieved some success, although not perfect performance, on simple auditory comprehension tasks. The verbal and gestural output tasks, on the other hand, were so difficult for him that he would consistently fail if we were to use them as treatment tasks. Second, research findings on the recovery patterns of individuals with left hemisphere damage obtained through use of the PICA suggested we could not expect functional changes to occur on verbal or gestural output tasks until auditory comprehension skills improved.

We structured our auditory comprehension drills using communication books. The first communication book consisted of photographs taken with an instant camera which were displayed in a conventional three-ring binder. Photographs included those of family members and selected rehabilitation staff members as well as frequent health care, self care, and recreational activities. Initially, the pictures were presented three on a page to reduce confusion. In time Dallas effectively responded to eight pictures per page. In addition, the rehabilitation staff were instructed to speak with Dallas about treatment activities as well as point to activities in the book to assist his comprehension. Although initially the book was designed to augment Dallas's ability to understand and respond to his partner's questions and instructions, he was encouraged to use the book to express his personal needs.

Almost immediately, the limitations of the communication book, as described above, became apparent. Therefore, Dallas's family was asked to bring photograph albums from home depicting family activities, familiar locations, and so forth. In addition, the family brought in a portfolio with several of Dallas's design accomplishments. The photographs in the portfolio were reorganized such that a picture showing an overall view was included along with photos of aspects of the projects. Within just a few days, Dallas used these work-related photos to augment his attempts at conversation (Fig. 12–1). As an additional assist, Dallas's wife wrote a 10 page biography about her husband's life. With this background information, staff members were able to supplement Dallas's efforts to communicate using the communication books, limited gestures, and increasingly consistent yes-no responses (head nodding).

The next phase of intervention was to improve Dallas's reading skills. Reading recognition was a primary focus, because reading skills would permit the use of a more compact, complete communication augmentation book. Printed words were included under each of the photographs in Dallas's expanding photographic communication books. Daily, Dallas would practice reading the printed word and identifying the corresponding photograph. When he was able to recognize a word consistently, the photograph was removed from the book and for 1 week an attempt was made to have him use the word only without the accompanying photograph. Later, the daily communication augmentation book was reduced to a 5 by 8 inch notebook containing only words and no photographs. At its largest, the communication book was 30 pages long, with 17 different categories of messages, including people, places, personal needs, medical messages, months and days, numbers, and the alphabet.

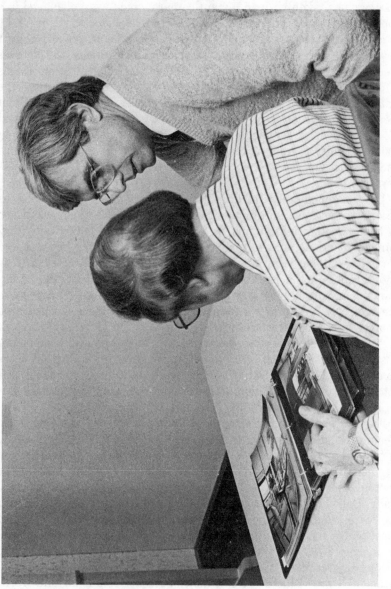

Figure 12–1. Dallas and his speech-language clinician using the communication book.

Gestures. As Dallas's health stabilized, he began to use gestures. However, initially only one gesture was easily recognized by the staff— palm up for "I don't know." Other gestures used naturally appeared to have no consistent meaning. An attempt was made to teach specific gestures from standard gestural systems. This was almost completely unsuccessful, at least partially as a result of limb apraxia, which made it difficult for Dallas to learn new, motorically complex gestures. We took a somewhat different approach in our effort to establish a repertoire of gestures. The help of family and staff was elicited to observe and document the gestural patterns produced by Dallas in natural communication situations. When Dallas produced a propositional gesture, an attempt would be made to attach a specific meaning to it. Using this approach, over the months of his recovery, Dallas developed a broad repertoire of meaningful gestures. These gestures were recognizable by minimally trained partners.

By 9 months following his CVA, Dallas's communication efforts were augmented by three systems: the communication book, related to specific communication needs, the more general conversational photograph book, and a repertoire of gestures. Table 12–1 illustrates results of the PICA, which was administered seven times during the first year. A review of this table suggests by the 9 months, overall performance had increased from the 22nd to the 50th percentile. At this time, he was responding accurately and appropriately to yes-no questions with head nods and shakes to indicate yes and no and with gestures to indicate "I don't know," "maybe," and "Your question is going in the wrong direction, ask something else."

Speech. With some basic aspects of communication augmentation in place, a program of intervention focusing on improving verbal output was begun at approximately 9 months following onset. Melodic Intonation Therapy (Sparks and Holland, 1976) is a highly structured, four level program in which natural melody patterns are used to

Table 12–1. PICA results (in percentile rankings) During the First Year Following Cerebrovascular Accident

MAO	Overall	Gestural	Verbal	Graphic
1	22	20	10	39
4	37	45	13	61
5	42	71	22	56
6	45	70	36	50
7	51	71	37	66
8	50	67	33	73
11	54	79	41	63

facilitate speech. Dallas appeared to be a good candidate for this approach because of his improving auditory comprehension skills and his good error recognition skills in the presence of continued poor ability to repeat words and phrases. The program involves selection of everyday words and phrases and identifying a natural melody for each phrase. Dallas was first taught to imitate the melody only, and then to imitate the words and melody along with the clinician. Gradually both the melody and the clinician's stimulus were faded. Using this approach, Dallas's verbal repertoire gradually began to expand, until he was able to produce 35 to 40 different words and phrases in the treatment session and at home.

Phase II. Transition to the Community

Throughout his recovery, Dallas demonstrated a strong interest in returning to work in some capacity. However, Dallas and his wife had closed his business during his hospitalization because they realized that the business could not operate successfully without his fulltime participation. In preparation for the phase of intervention that focused on return to work, another needs assessment was completed (Table 12-2). Dallas's mandatory need for communication in a variety of locations with strangers, clients, business associates, and family members was clearly reflected in these results.

Table 12-2. Dallas's List of Mandatory Communication Needs

Locations and Positions
   Throughout his home
   Throughout the design center
   In client homes and businesses

Communication Partners
   Family members
   Clients
   Strangers
   Several persons at a time
   Person unfamiliar with system

Message Needs
   Call attention
   Answer yes-no questions
   Make standard requests
   Provide unique information
   Carry on conversation
   Express emotion
   Express esthetic opinion
   Greet people

In preparation for Dallas's return to professional activity, most of his design materials were moved to a single room in his home, which was modified into a studio with extensive wall shelving. The goal was to provide him with a communication augmentation aid—his studio with catalogs, paint samples, carpet samples, tile chips, and so forth—easily available to him. When in this room, he would be able to indicate a wide variety of messages related to the specifics of interior design.

In addition to the studio, Dallas continued his pre-CVA involvement in the Seattle Design Center, a large complex of interior design-related stores and shops where Dallas could take his clients and together go from shop to shop to view options and finalize their plans. Several months after his discharge from the rehabilitation center, Dallas invited a young artist to join him as an assistant. With Dallas participating as best he could, the artist drove, interviewed the clients, made drawings for proposals, made appointments, and so forth. Gradually, some of Dallas's former customers began to return to him for additional work on their homes and small businesses. Observation of Dallas and his assistant with clients revealed how well Dallas maximized his communication effectiveness with his limited communication skills. However, the communication limitations were very apparent, as Dallas spoke approximately 10 different words during interactions with his clients.

A speech-language pathologist from our center was actively involved with Dallas and his assistant as they learned to communicate together. The assistant was familiarized with Dallas's communication tools, the communication book, the portfolio, and the home studio. Also, Dallas and his assistant were acompanied on visits to the Design Center with clients. Gradually, Dallas and his assistant developed a system of shared knowledge, gestures, speech, and communication tools described earlier, which supported a productive working relationship.

Phase III. A Portable Speech System

Regular speech treatment did not continue after Dallas returned to work. We saw him periodically to check on his progress. During these visits, changing communication needs were reviewed. The need to speak a greater number of words and phrases intelligibly and quickly was apparent. The communication books, the studio, and the design center provided a good deal of communication support; however, the process of decision making between client and designer required additional interpersonal communication ability. The augmentation approaches that were in place allowed Dallas to communicate a relatively large number of "content messages," including names, places, nouns, and adjectives related to interior design. Dallas and his communication partners appeared to need conversational management phrases that would allow Dallas to control the decision-making conversations that are critical to his work. A screening of Dallas's capabilities revealed that while his reading recognition skills had improved considerably, his spelling skills remained severely impaired. He was able to select only the first letter of some words, but was unable to spell spontaneously any of the words he needed to communicate.

System Selection.   Because the needs assessment indicated that a portable speech output system was required, Dallas was given a brief trial using a Handivoice 110 communicator, a portable speech synthesis unit on which the user directly selects messages (HC Electronics, Mill Valley, California). The system is factory programmed with words and phrases, but unique messages may be created by entering them sound by sound. Dallas demonstrated the ability to read the small print on the control display, and he could understand the multilevel system for retrieving messages. He was able to select messages from the four colored displays. He learned to erase the memory and repeat a message. However, during the 1 week trial, he did not learn to formulate messages that required more than one entry. The decision was made to not to purchase the Handivoice 110 at that time, because the vocabulary offered to Dallas was too limited. The Handivoice 110 was not field programmable, so most of the words related to the field of interior design that Dallas needed were not available to him on the unit. For 3 years Dallas continued to use the communication systems described previously.

When the Handivoice 130 (Fig. 12–2) was introduced in 1983 with one level of field programmable memory, Dallas along with his Division of Vocational Rehabilitation (DVR) counselor, was familiarized with the device. Dallas demonstrated the ability to perform the same functions that he had learned earlier on the Handivoice 110. With this information a formal request was made to DVR for purchase of the system. After reopening Dallas's case, DVR agreed to such a purchase.

Training.   Dallas, his wife, and his business assistant came to our center for instructional sessions. They were introduced to the Handivoice 130. Dallas's wife and his business assistant learned to program the fifth level of memory with messages appropriate to the business. Each of them proposed messages to be programmed into the Handivoice 130. As they observed their business-related interaction, they noted messages that might enhance communication effectiveness. At the end of 2 weeks, Dallas reviewed the list of proposed messages

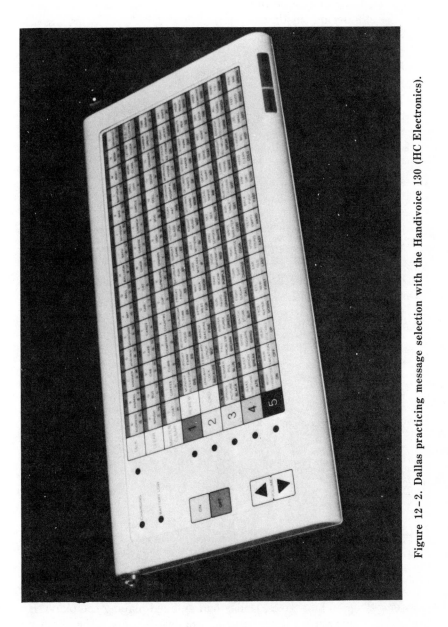

Figure 12–2. Dallas practicing message selection with the Handivoice 130 (HC Electronics).

and chose those that he preferred to have stored in the system. These messages are listed below, with an occasional explanatory note.

1. This is going to be fun.
2. Let's decide this later.
3. Let's move on.
4. When will that be done?
5. Let's get this moving.
6. Please say that again.
7. I did not hear you.
8. When will we meet again?
9. I would like to speak to Adrienne (to call his wife at her work)
10. Have Adrienne call home.
11. Contract
12. Drawings
13. Model
14. Proposal
15. Arise Center (a project Dallas on which Dallas was working)
16. Cornish (an Art Institute where Dallas worked with design students regarding the design needs of disabled individuals)

Other messages were already programmed in the Handivoice 130 and were highlighted for Dallas's use.

1. How are you?
2. I am fine
3. Thank you
4. Maybe
5. Table
6. Chair
7. Elevator
8. Appointment
9. Circle
10. Church
11. Lunch
12. Dinner
13. Bed
14. Who
15. Where
16. What

During the 2 week period when the proposed message list was being developed, Dallas practiced the control aspects of the communication system. Prior to his stroke, Dallas had enjoyed playing the piano. He referred to this period of practice as "finger exercises." There was no attempt to use the system for communication, only to develop efficiency in operating it.

After the initial list of messages was stored or highlighted, Dallas was familiarized with a gradually expanding number of words and phrases on the device. Dallas's message retrieval training program was based on sets of 10 words and phrases. The master overlay for the Handivoice 130 was visually too complex for Dallas. We used the blue overlay, which contained many nouns, and then highlighted field programmed messages (level 5) and interpersonal message (level 1) on the blue overlay (Fig. 12–3) using stickers. After Dallas demonstrated the ability to select 7 of 10 messages, the next set of 10 messages was introduced.

After Dallas became familiar with the first set of 10 messages, he was encouraged to bring the communication system with him to working sessions with his assistant and clients. He was instructed only to use the system when he was "stuck" and knew that a message on the system would resolve the communication breakdown. After approximately 2 weeks of using the Handivoice 130 in this restricted manner, Dallas's assistant reported that he was beginning to use the system much more frequently. He selected "favorite" messages promptly and appropriately. Occasionally, the assistant would suggest that he use additional phrases in particular situations. Each evening, he would practice with the system for about half an hour. At the time this chapter was written, Dallas had used the Handivoice 130 for

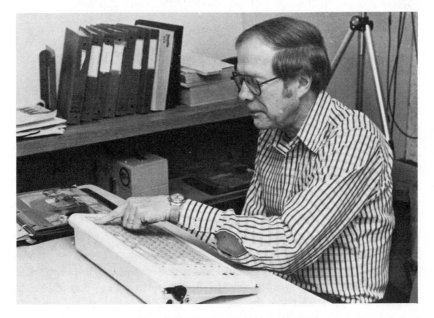

Figure 12–3. The Handivoice 130.

8 weeks. We were increasing the number of messages that he could retrieve by about 10 message every 2 weeks.

Dallas takes the Handivoice 130 with him to all business interactions. He usually has it available to him in social situations as well. At this time, he does not formulate grammatically complete sentences by selecting several words or phrases. Rather, he tends to communicate a message by retrieving a single word or phrase. At times he prefers to have a single word rather than a phrase stored in the system, because he can introduce a topic with a single word and then convey his preferred message through speech or gesture. At one point Dallas indicated that he wished to be able to retrieve the word "lunch." We offered to program the message, "Shall we go to lunch?" or "Do you want to go to lunch?" Dallas rejected both of these suggestions, preferring the single word "lunch." He then retrieved "lunch" with the Handivoice 130 and gestured with hand and facial movements a very positive response. Next, he retrieved "lunch" and raised his eyebrows as if to ask whether or not his listener might be interested in going to lunch. Finally, he retrieved the word "lunch" a third time and gestured the "thumbs down" signal, as if to say, "Of course, I'm not interested in lunch." For several years Dallas has communicated with minimal speech and he had learned numerous effective communication strategies, which he is now combining with the capabilities of the Handivoice 130. Obviously, Dallas's integration of the Handivoice system into his total communication approach will take years.

QUESTIONS FOR THE CLINICIAN

Question 1. Does Dallas speak more frequently now that he has a communication augmentation system that produces synthesized speech?

Yes, he frequently says words immediately after they are spoken by the system. When he is alone practicing with the system, he imitates almost every phrase as clearly as he can. When he uses the system as a communication aid with strangers, he does not imitate the messages as frequently as when he is alone.

The potential effects of synthesized speech output on the recovery of severely apraxic or aphasic individuals have not yet been studied systematically. However, clinicians are beginning to document some very intriguing cases. For example, Warren and Datta (1981) reported the case of a severely head-injured individual with a diagnosis of severe nonfluent aphasia who was trained to use a Handivoice 110. This patient was seen 4½ years following the injury and was trained to formulate complete messages word by word using the system. Although the patient's condition was considered stable when the system was introduced, verbal communication began to appear after only a short period of system use. As systems become more available clinically, the impact of synthesized speech as feedback to the nonspeaking patient will be important to investigate.

Question 2. Do you feel that a system such as the Handivoice 130 is a useful communication augmentation system for all aphasic adults? What other communication augmentation devices have been used successfully with adult aphasics?

The Handivoice system is *not* the answer for all aphasic individuals. Recall that aphasia is a language disorder which impairs the ability to interpret and formulate symbolic information and usually crosses all language modalities. The aphasic individual will have difficulty not only with listening and speaking but also with reading and writing. Dallas's aphasia was considered moderate at the time the Handivoice 130 was recommended. His inability to produce understandable speech was the result, to a large extent, of his apraxia of speech.

Certain user capabilities are necessary for successful operation of the Handivoice 130. Reading recognition is required to select the messages to be produced by the device. Visual discrimination to locate the preferred message on the control display is essential. In addition, good motor control is required to depress the appropriate location of the direct selection control interface. Lastly, reduced ability to string messages (words or phrases) together into grammatical sequences might also limit the usefulness of this system for large number of aphasic individuals. Many of these capabilities are beyond the level of severely aphasic individuals.

In addition to the capabilities described above, the individual's communication needs must be considered when selecting the Handivoice 130. The ability to select messages that will communicate the desired content must be demonstrated. For Dallas, conversational control and a specific number of work-related messages were important. Conversational control refers to the individual's ability to direct conversational interactions. Speech output is a very effective means for communicating conversational control messages because a relatively small number of intelligible and rapidly retrieved phrases is required. For another aphasic individual with more limited social and vocational contacts and with very familiar communication partners, the Handivoice 130 might not assist effectively in the communication of the unique messages that adults often wish to express.

At the time this book was written, the communication augmentation interventions for aphasic individuals are limited to communication books and boards, gestures or restricted signing, and residual writing. Occasionally, applications of electronic communication approaches are appearing in the literature, and they are presented in the *Additional Readings* list at the end of this chapter. To date, the aphasic nonspeaking individual has not received the attention from the communication augmentation field that other groups, such as the physically handicapped have received. It is hoped this will change.

Question 3.   Are gestural approaches more appropriate for aphasic individuals than those that rely on communication devices?

In Chapter 9, we discussed in depth the issues which are critical in the use of gestural approaches for communication augmentation. When considering aphasic individuals in particular, these issues generally revolve around two questions: Does the individual have the ability to use the gestural approach? Do the gestures meet the individual's communication needs?

We have already discussed the deficits in aphasic individuals that may interfere with successful use of a system like the Handivoice 130. These same deficits may preclude the successful use of a gestural approach to communication. There is a growing body of literature (see *Additional Readings*) that documents the presence of gestural deficits in aphasic individuals. This finding is not surprising if you consider the fundamental similarities between verbal and gestural communication. Both have a symbolic component, relying on arbitrary relationships between the words or gestures and the meaning expressed, and both rely on complex sequences of movements. Deficits in language, cognition, or motor control may preclude the use of such approaches as a primary means of communication.

We must also consider whether a particular gestural approach meets the communication needs of the individual. First, we need to know some things about the individual's communication partners. Are there only a few potential partners? Do they already know a sign or gestural system? Is it reasonable to expect them to learn such a system? Or does the aphasic individual need to communicate with people who are unfamiliar with the gestures? Second, we need to determine the types of messages the individual is likely to express. Does the aphasic individual need to direct caregivers or are self-care activities performed independently? For example, could the individual use a gesture to indicate thirst in order to get some water, or is the individual able to get up and get some water independently? Does the individual need to express more abstract and complex concepts? If so, can the gestural approach under consideration meet those needs?

With these words of caution about selecting a gestural approach, it is apparent that gestures are not an easy substitute for speech in severely aphasic individuals. In fact, there are a wide range of deficits that may limit an aphasic individual's ability to use gestures. However, it would be misleading to conclude that all gestural approaches should be abandoned for aphasic patients. It is no more appropriate to abandon the gestural mode on the basis of gestural deficits than it is to abandon the verbal modality because of speech or language deficits. Carefully selected gestures may be used by aphasic individuals to convey some messages. Other gestures may be used profitably to supplement speech attempts. Dallas's use of multiple modes of communication illustrates a successful integration of a number of different communication approaches. It is important that we do not neglect a channel of communication that efficiently serves even a limited number of communication needs.

ACKNOWLEDGMENT

We wish to thank Marilyn Morro, an occupational therapist at our center, who assisted Dallas in organizing his return to work.

REFERENCES

Porch, B. E. *Porch Index of Communicative Ability*. Palo Alto, CA: Consulting Psychologists Press, 1967.

Raven, J. C. *Guide to the standard progressive matrices*. London: H. K. Lewis, 1960.

Sparks, R., and Holland, A. Method: Melodic Intonation Therapy for aphasia. *Journal of Speech and Hearing Disorders*, 1976, *41*, 287–297.

Warren, R. L., and Datta, K. D. The return of speech 4½ years post head injury: A case report. In R. Brookshire (Ed.), *Clinical Aphasiology Conference Proceedings*. Minneapolis, MN: BRK Publishers, 1981, pp. 301–308.

Wechsler, D. *Wechsler Adult Intelligence Scale manual*. New York: Psychological Corporation, 1955.

ADDITIONAL READINGS

Anderson, T. P. Rehabilitation of patients with completed stroke. In F. Kottke, J. Stillwell, and J. Lehmann (Eds.), *Krusen's handbook of physical medicine and rehabilitation*. Philadelphia: W. B. Saunders, 1982, pp. 679–690.

Bugbee, J. K., and Hanecak, J. Developing a communication board for the aphasic adult. *ASHA*, 1980, *22*, 684.

Cicone, M., Wapner, W., Foldi, N., Zurif, E., and Gardner, H. The relationship between gesture and language in aphasic communication. *Brain and Language*, 1979, *8*, 324–349.

Daniloff, J. K., Noll, J. D., Fristoe, M., and Lloyd, L. L. Gesture recognition in patients with aphasia. *Journal of Speech and Hearing Disorders*, 1982, *47*, 43–47.

Davis, S., Artes, R., and Hoops, R. Verbal expression and expressive pantomine in aphasic patients. In Lebrun and R. Hoops (Ed.), *Problems of aphasia*, Lisse: Swets and Zeitliyer B. V., 1979.

Dowden, P. A., Marshall, R. C., and Tompkins, C. A. Amer-Ind sign as a communicative facilitator for aphasic and apraxic patients. In R. Brookshire (Ed.), *Clinical Aphasiology Conference Proceedings*. Minneapolis, MN: BRK Publishers, 1981, pp. 133–140.

Duffy, R. J., and Buck, R. A. A study of the relationship between propositional (pantomime) and subpropositional (facial expression) extraverbal behaviors in aphasics. *Folio Phoniatrica*, 1979, *31*, 129–136.

Duffy, R. J. and Duffy, J. R. Three studies of deficits in pantomimic expression and pantomimic recognition in aphasia. *Journal of Speech and Hearing Research*, 1981, *24*, 70–34.

Eagleson, H. M., Vaughan, G. R., and Knudson, A. B. C. Hand signals for dysphasia. *Archives of Physical Medicine and Rehabilitation*, 1970, *51*, 111–113.

Fristoe, M., and Lloyd, L. L. Planning an initial expressive sign lexicon for persons with severe communication impairment. *Journal of Speech and Hearing Disorders*, 1980, *45*, 170–180.

Gianotti, G., and Lemmo, M. A. Comprehension of symbolic gestures in aphasia. *Brain and Language*, 1976, *3*, 451–460.

Glass, A. V., Gazzaniga, M. S., and Premack, D. Artifical language training in global aphasics. *Neuropsychologia*, 1973, *11*, 95–103.

Goodglass, H., and Kaplan, E. Disturbances of gesture and pantomime in aphasia. *Brain*, 1963, *86*, 703–720.

Katz, R. C. Using microcomputers in the diagnosis and treatment of chronic aphasic adults. *Seminars in Speech and Language*, 1984, *5*, 11–22.

Katz, R. C. A computerized treatment system for chronic aphasic patients. In R. Brookshire (Ed.), *Clinical Aphasiology Conference Proceedings*. Minneapolis, MN: BRK Publishers, 1983.

Katz, R., LaPointe, L., and Markel, N. Coverbal behavior and aphasic speakers. In R. Brookshire (Ed.), *Clinical Aphasiology Conference Proceedings*. Minneapolis, MN: BRK Publishers, 1978, pp. 164–173.

Kimura, D. The neurological basis of language qua gesture. In H. Whitaker and H. A. Whitaker (Eds.), *Studies in neurolinguistics* (Vol. 2). New York: Academic Press, 1976.

Kirschner, H., and Webb, W. Selective involvement of the auditory — verbal modality in an acquired communication disorder: Benefit from sign language therapy. *Brain and Language*, 1981, *13*, 161–170.

Kohl, F. Effects of motoric requirements on the acquisition of manual sign responses by severely handicapped students. *American Journal of Mental Deficiency*, 1981, *85*(4), 396–403.

Peterson, L., and Kirshner, H. Gestural impairment and gestural ability in aphasia: A review. *Brain and Language*, 1981, *14*, 333–348.

Pickett, L. An assessment of gestural and pantomime deficits in aphasic population. *Acta Symbolica*, 1974, *5*(3), 69–86.

Rao, P. R., and Horner, J. Gesture as a deblocking modality in a severe aphasic patient. In R. Brookshire (Ed.), *Clinical Aphasiology Conference Proceedings*, Minneapolis, MN: BRK Publishers, 1978, pp. 180–187.

Schlanger, P. H., and Frieman, R. Pantomime therapy with aphasics. *Aphasia-Apraxia-Agnosia*, 1979, *1*(2), 34–39.

Shane, H. C., and Wilber, R. B. Prediction of experience sign potential based on motor control. *Sign Language Studies*, 1980, Winter, pp. 331–348.

Yorkston, K. M., and Dowden, P. A. Nonspeech language and communication systems. In A. Holland (Ed.), *Language disorder in adults*. San Diego, CA: College-Hill Press, 1984.

CHAPTER 13

Rhonda

Etiology: Developmental delay and cerebral palsy
Onset: Congenital
Approach: Unicorn Keyboard with Talking Word Board Program
Focus: We present the case of a developmentally delayed woman with cerebral palsy, unable to read because of her limited education. We discuss the issues of symbol selection for nonreaders.

BACKGROUND

Rhonda is a 22 year old woman with significant cognitive deficits and spastic quadriplegia secondary to an anoxic episode at birth. She has lived all of her life in her parents' home, where she is cared for by an attendant. Schooling was limited to three years at a local school for the retarded, where she was taught some limited signing.

Rhonda ambulates by means of a manual wheelchair, which she propels with her left foot. According to her attendant, she usually propels the chair backwards rather than forward because she "gets better traction." She is dependent in all activities of daily living (ADLs). Specifically, she needs complete assistance in dressing owing to her poor motor control, her poor planning, and her visual-spatial deficits. She can feed herself with assistance in cutting the food and steadying the utensil. Transfers from the wheelchair to the toilet or bed require nearly complete support from the attendant. Medically, Rhonda has few problems. She had had some seizures as a child, but these are completely controlled by phenobarbital at this time.

Communication has been a significant problem for Rhonda and her attendant for many years. Rhonda's speech is severely dysarthric, resulting in only four distinguishable words: "yes," "Mom," "ball," and "ow." Some additional concepts, for example, "no" and "dog," are conveyed through gestures, pointing, and modified signing. Rhonda has had no formal training in symbol or word recognition, although the attendant did train her in spelling on an electric typewriter. In three years of training, Rhonda learned to type to dictation approximately 50 words, such as "boat" and "dog."

Rhonda was referred to our center by the attendant who had been training her in spelling. He believed that the typewriter was not a viable system for Rhonda because her typing was too slow and her vocabulary too limited. He also believed that she had become increasingly frustrated by her inability to express herself. This frustration had brought Rhonda to tears when she could not convey her thoughts and needs. Her few signs and words simply could not adequately meet her communication needs.

These concerns were heightened by the fact that Rhonda's parents had recently developed some major medical problems. Rhonda's caregivers began to recognize the possibility that she may have to move from her parent's house to a home for the disabled. There was concern that few people in the home would understand Rhonda's signs or her speech. In addition, they may not have time to use the "twenty questions" approach to know what she wanted to express. Everyone believed it was essential for her to become a more independent communicator.

INITIAL EVALUATION

Communication Needs Assessment

The concerns just described contributed to our assessment of Rhonda's communication needs. Through additional questioning of the attendant and Rhonda's parents, we established a list of communication needs for her (Table 13–1). The list showed that Rhonda needed a portable communication system with speech output.

Ideally, the system would permit her to communicate unique and unpredictable information.

Capability Assessment

Motor Control.   Rhonda was first seen at our center when she was 20 years old. In the motor control evaluation, we first examined her upper extremity control. It appeared that finger control, in general, was insufficient for the complex motor movements of sign, although she was able to make some clear signs using the entire hand. Control of her right index finger was sufficient, however, for her to activate any keys larger than 0.5 inch across, regardless of the range of excursion required in activation. The range of Rhonda's arm movement

Table 13-1. Specific Needs Statements for Rhonda

Communication Partners

M   Someone who cannot read (e.g., fellow residents
     at a home for the disabled)
M   Someone who has limited time or patience
M   Several people at one time
M   Someone who is unfamiliar with the system
D   Someone who is across the room or in another room
D   Some strangers

Locations

M   Sitting in her wheelchair
M   Lying in her bed
M   Sitting in bed
D   In a dark room
M   In a bright room
D   In a noisy room
M   In a quiet room
M   In a variety of rooms (at home or in a facility)
M   Moving from room to room
M   In a van or car
D   Outdoors

Message Needs

M   Call attention
M   Make requests
M   Answer yes/no questions
M   Express emotion
M   Carry on a conversation
M   Give her opinion
M   Signal emergencies
M   Convey basic self-care needs
M   Greet people
D   Relate unique events
D   Provide unique information

Key: M = Mandatory
     D = Desirable but not mandatory

was not limiting in that it was sufficient for her to activate keys anywhere on her rather large laptray. These results suggested that Rhonda had sufficient motor control to use a variety of communication approaches by means of direct selection. No additional motor evaluation was necessary at that time.

Cognition and Language. Rhonda's cognitive abilities had been tested on several occasions. However, her family did not release the information to us because they felt strongly that the scores did not reflect her true capabilities. The family expressed concern that our recommendations would be biased by the low scores.

We then turned to an assessment of Rhonda's linguistic capabilities.

Screening demonstrated that Rhonda's reading ability was too low for formal evaluation by means of standardized testing. In informal assessment Rhonda was able to identify 3 of 10 highly egocentric words: "Rhonda," "dog," and "Mom." The attendant demonstrated Rhonda's spelling by having her type words she had learned to type to dictation. She was able to type 8 of 12 such words at a rate of 1.5 words/minute. Because she was able to activate the typewriter keys rapidly, this slow rate could not be attributed to motor deficits, but rather it reflected linguistic and cognitive processing time. It is important to note that Rhonda was not able to recognize seven of the eight words she had typed, nor was she able to match any pictures to those words. Her typing appeared to be stimulus dependent.

We screened Rhonda's ability to recognize graphic symbols of increasing abstractness. She was able to point to photographs of common objects with 100% reliability, whether given the name of the object or a question relating to it. When we changed from photographs to line drawings, Rhonda's accuracy dropped to 80%. However, we found that this accuracy improved with very brief training in recognition of the line drawings. In this evaluation, we could not address all issues related to symbol selection and display. The remaining issues were deferred until the intervention phase.

Recommendations

At the conclusion of this evaluation, it was clear that Rhonda had sufficient motor control to activate keys on almost any type of keyboard. However, she clearly did not have the linguistic abilities to communicate by selecting letters, words, or phrases. Her spelling and word recognition were too limited for all of her message needs. Rhonda would have to use a less abstract symbol system, preferably one which did not require a great deal of training.

For these reasons, following this first evaluation in 1982, we advised the family against any commercially available communication devices. We recommended that a communication board be designed that could be mounted onto her wheelchair laptray. The board was to be constructed so that the symbols used could be changed as we came to know Rhonda's symbol comprehension and as her communication needs were clarified. We recommended further that the board have the capacity for multiple displays for different communication environments, if Rhonda could learn to handle several different communication overlays.

This communication board clearly would not meet all of Rhonda's communication needs. For example, it would not provide her with a means of communicating with partners across the room or in another room. It would not allow her to communicate while in a dimly lit room. She could not talk with anyone who could not look at her board—for example, the driver of a vehicle or anyone who might be too busy when she wanted to communicate. The board itself would not provide her with a means of calling attention or signaling an emergency; Rhonda would have to be taught to use speech or a bell for this. Depending on the number of items Rhonda could handle on the display, the board may or may not provide her with a means to relate information about some unique events in her rather limited life.

In our opinion, there was no approach which could meet all of Rhonda's communication needs at that time. We considered it essential that Rhonda begin to use communication boards to expand her understanding and use of expressive communication. There was no justification for waiting for a "better" system to appear on the market because Rhonda could clearly benefit immediately from the presently available boards.

However, Rhonda's family held a different opinion. They expressed concern that such a board would limit the number of messages she could convey. It would not allow her to communicate "all the things she wants to say." In addition, they felt that she needed a system with speech output, so she could "be a normal speaker." They decided to postpone the development of any new communication approach until it was possible to meet all of Rhonda's communication needs. In the meantime, they would prefer to continue with their current system of "twenty questions," some signs, and some words.

INTERVENTION

System Selection

Nearly 2 years after the first evaluation, a system that would meet many of Rhonda's and her parents' needs became available commercially. The system comprised several components: the Unicorn Keyboard, manufactured by Unicorn Engineering (Oakland, California), the Adaptive Firmware Card and Talking Word Board Program of Adaptive Peripherals (Seattle, Washington), and an Apple II+ or IIe computer. Together these components constituted what we will call the Talking Word Board system. It provides a field programmable membrane keyboard onto which one can place a fully customized set of display symbols. This keyboard, with 128 keys, is shown in Figure 13-1. The system permits printed output via the computer screen; the addition of an Echo II Speech Synthesizer, available from Street Electronics (Carpinteria, California), provides the speech output.

The remarkable feature of this system is the extent to which most of its functions can be fully customized for the individual. First, the board and the keys are large enough to permit the use of any type of symbol system, from photographs to single words or letters. Although the actual size of the keys cannot be changed, the same message can be programmed "behind" several adjacent keys to accommodate large pictures or symbols. Second, the messages retrieved with each key activation can be completely individualized, ranging in length from a single number or letter to an utterance of up to 40 characters. This allows us to use the keyboard most efficiently to meet the individual's specific message needs. A third advantage in this respect is that the system has up to nine levels of memory associated with each key, and additional "vocabularies" can be stored on a disk and programmed into the board at the touch of a key. This permits much greater flexibility in the messages and the overlays. For example, one user might use all nine levels at all times, changing levels independently. Another user might use one level and overlay in one environment, and another level and overlay in another setting.

A fourth advantage of this system is that, when used with the Firmware Card, the responsiveness of the membrane keys can be selected for the individual. The keys can be set to activate immediately upon contact, or after a longer period of time, such as several seconds. This permits users to slide their hands along the keyboard without

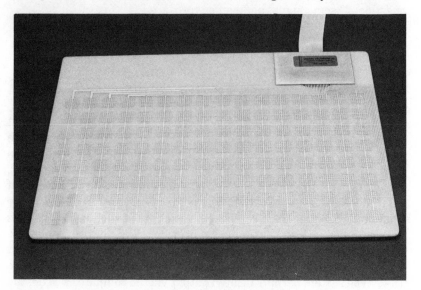

Figure 13-1. Unicorn keyboard.

activating keys inadvertently. The proper setting depends on the individual's motor and cognitive capabilities.

We brought Rhonda back to the center for a trial with the Talking Word Board. At our request, Rhonda's parents brought a number of photographs and pictures that were of particular importance to her. We made a simple overlay with these pictures, some line drawings, more abstract symbols, and some words. Then we demonstrated the board for Rhonda by pressing her finger onto the photograph of her mother. The system responded immediately with "Mom, come here," and Rhonda smiled broadly.

We stepped Rhonda through the other pictures and symbols, including one item that was a yellow card with her name. We practiced all of the items by telling her to "press the picture of the _____" or "Press the one with your name." Then we let Rhonda play with the system for a few minutes while we discussed appropriate symbols for her overlays. When we turned to Rhonda again, we chose to give her a quick test with a more difficult request. I told her I'd forgotten her name, and she immediately responded by pressing the yellow card. She was all smiles when the system responded: "My name is Rhonda."

This system was the first step in the development of a system for Rhonda that would provide her with all the advantages of a customized communication board as described earlier. In addition, it would provide printed and speech output. This would permit her to communicate with partners who were unfamiliar with her system because they would need to understand only the output, not Rhonda's display symbols. In addition, Rhonda would be able to communicate rapidly and from a distance with partners who have limited time and patience, or partners who are unable to look at her board. Furthermore, the system would provide Rhonda with immediate feedback regarding her selection.

There was a significant disadvantage to the current system, however. It is clearly too bulky to be mounted to a wheelchair. For this reason, the system as it was could only be used for training or for communication in a single setting. Nonetheless, we recommended that the system be purchased and training proceed. We would meanwhile work with several commercial software businesses to interface the Unicorn to a portable computer, such as the Epson HX-20.

Symbol Selection

In recommending the specific symbols to be used for an individual, we usually work from a hierarchy of symbols, as shown in Figure 13-2. This chart shows some representative graphic symbol systems ranked according to the symbolic load or level of abstraction of the symbols. This load can range from a completely arbitrary relationship between the symbol and its referent, as in the printed word, to a one-to-one referential relationship, as exists between a photograph of an object and the object itself. Other types of symbols are better described as iconic, bearing a more universally accepted meaning, for example an up-turned arrow to mean "up." For a more complete discussion of symbol systems, the reader should refer to the references listed in the *References* and the *Additional Readings* sections of this chapter.

It is essential for several reasons that we consider the symbolic load of each symbol used on the control display of a communication system. First, the user must learn the symbol and be able to recognize it reliably, even under the pressure of communication. Several studies (Clark, 1981; Hughes, 1979) have shown that abstract symbols are more difficult to learn and retain than concrete symbols. This may be especially true for nonspeaking individuals with language impairments or learning disabilities. It may be more effective to limit the symbolic load of the symbols used, wherever possible.

A second reason for considering the symbolic load is related to the needs of the communication partner. First, we must know whether the communication partners need to utilize the display symbols in interpreting the speaker's message. For example, in some communication systems, the symbols selected by the user are transformed into other output for the listener. The Handivoice 130 is an example of this in that the user selects printed words or phrases

Symbol System	Relationship to Referent	Examples #1	#2
1. Printed word	Arbitrary	"building"	"this"
2. Blissymbols	Arbitrary or Iconic	------ △	/ ------
3. Picsyms or Line drawings	Iconic	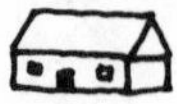 🏠	(Drawing not possible)
4. Photographs	Referential	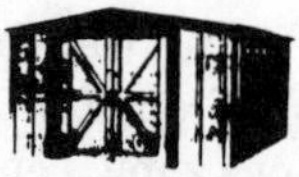 🏗	(Photo not possible)

Figure 13–2. Hierarchy of symbol systems. Blissymbols ©1979 by Blissymbolics Communication Institute, Toronto, Ontario, Canada. Used with permission.

from a display, but the output is synthesized speech. When such systems are used, then, there is no need to consider the intelligibility of the symbols to the communication partners; they simply do not need to understand those symbols.

However, in some cases the symbols serve both users and partners, for control display and for output. In selecting a symbol system for these approaches it is essential that we consider the intelligibility of the symbol system to the communication partners. Musselwhite (1982) examined the intelligibility (or "transparency") of three symbol systems: Blissymbolics, Picsyms, and Rebus. She found that Blissymbols were significantly less intelligible to untrained viewers than were Picsyms or Rebus symbols. If the symbols must be understood by a broad audience of untrained partners, we must consider the feasibility of using printed words next to each symbol. If the nonspeaking individual has any nonreading partners, this use of words will not suffice, and we must limit the symbolic load of the symbols (Musselwhite, 1983).

A third reason to consider symbolic load is related to the lexical limitations of the system, its potential for conveying all messages. The symbol systems shown in Figure 13-2 vary greatly in the extent to which they can convey all concepts. For example, it is simply not possible to make a referential photograph of the concept "love." One can use an iconic symbol, such as a heart shape, or an arbitrary symbol. One could even use an *iconic* photograph, for example, a picture of a cherub, but this is a more abstract symbol, which must be learned. In general, the more abstract a symbol system is, the greater its potential for expressing unlimited concepts. English orthography and Blissymbolics are potentially unlimited in their lexicon, as long as both users and partners are familiar with the word or symbol convention used. The Picsyms and Rebus systems allow a somewhat more limited vocabulary (Musselwhite, 1983) unless the system is expanded to include arbitrary symbols which must be learned.

A final consideration in selecting symbols is the semantic flexibility of each symbol. For example, the word "home" can refer to a middle-class split-level house, a log cabin, or even a grass hut. A line drawing tends to narrow the range of concepts, however, because it resembles some homes but not others. A photograph narrows the field even further, leading the partner to think only of the specific home pictured.

Because of these considerations we do not automatically choose a single symbol system for an individual. Instead we use these factors to guide us in the selection of *each* symbol used for a concept. To develop a set of symbols for Rhonda, we began with a list of the concepts she needed to express. We asked the family to make a diary of everything that Rhonda communicated, by any modality, during a particular week. Table 13-2 shows an excerpt from this diary.

Table 13-2. Rhonda's Communication Diary

Date	Time	Idea expressed	How idea was conveyed
3/12	9 AM	No apple	Pushed the apple away
,,	,,	I want a banana	Pointed to banana
,,	,,	I want milk	Pointed to refrigerator; Mom asked yes/no questions
,,	,,	I want juice	Mom asked "Do you want more juice or more milk?"; she pointed to juice.
,,	9:30	I want to go outside	Wheeled to porch door and outside used her little cry to get attention; Mom asked yes/no questions.

This diary structured our approach in several respects. It gave a list of the concepts she tried to express throughout her typical day. It also showed which concepts she could already express independently, at least in this setting. For example, there was no need to give Rhonda a means of getting her listeners' attention; she did this effectively with her voice. In other settings, her "little cry" might not be effective or might not be socially acceptable, but in this setting it seemed appropriate.

Once we had determined what concepts Rhonda needed to express via the Talking Word Board, we then selected the appropriate symbols for the display. Using the hierarchy shown in Figure 13-2, we chose the highest level symbol she could recognize reliably for each concept. For example, Rhonda was able to recognize the printed word "Mom," so we did not need to use a Blissymbol, a line drawing, or a photograph for that concept; we could use the most space-saving symbol, the printed word. Because she did not recognize the word "toilet" but did recognize the concept in a line drawing and a photograph, we selected the line drawing because it is a higher level symbol and therefore more universally applicable. Rhonda did not recognize either the word or a line drawing of a grocery store, so we recommended that a photograph be used for that particular concept. In this way, we planned each symbol to be used on the Talking Word Board.

Training

Intervention goals were designed to move Rhonda as quickly as possible to functional use of the communication system. This necessitated that we group the symbols into categories, such as "food" and "recreation," and work with only a single category initially. We drilled Rhonda on the symbols, moving her through a hierarchy of tasks designed to familiarize her with the symbols and then demonstrate the power of the system in natural communication interactions. Table 13–3 shows the first five steps of this program.

Table 13–3. Program Hierarchy.

Task Level	Response Level	Variables
1. Identification of symbols	Pointing to one symbol	Symbol type, number, position, saliency; reinforcement; response time
2. Activation of symbol or key	Pressing one key	Key pressure, responsiveness; all of above
3. Naming objects shown	Pressing one key	Objects used, all of above
4. Single word response to narrow questions (e.g.What is your brother's name?)	Pressing one key	
5. Single word response to broader questions (e.g., What did you eat for lunch?)	Pressing one key	

During drills at levels 1 to 3, we made adjustments in several variables to maximize Rhonda's success. We manipulated the symbol types in terms of the symbolic load, usually decreasing the load of a symbol used because Rhonda's responses with it became unreliable as more demands were placed on her. We also manipulated the number of symbols, their position, their perceptual saliency and the type of reinforcement utilized. When Rhonda reached level 3 with the first group of symbols, we added a second group at levels 1 and 2.

Training at levels 3 and above was designed around the PACE format (see Chapter 9) in order to make the interactions more natural. At level 3 this meant that Rhonda was shown pictures of objects out of view of her attendant; she was to tell him which picture she saw. At levels 4 and 5, Rhonda was to answer questions about her life and activities or play games structured with her vocabulary. In all cases, the listener did not know the message to be communicated.

At the time this chapter was written, Rhonda was continuing this practice with single utterance responses, with a vocabulary of approximately 75 messages. The utterances were arranged on two overlays so that one met Rhonda's communication needs for the morning, with concepts related to eating breakfast and lunch, toileting, dressing, and therapies. The second overlay, changed by the attendant, served for afternoon and evening activities. Three weeks into the training program, Rhonda rarely initiated with the system, although she had always initiated with signs and vocalization. With reminders to "say it with the board," Rhonda was able to use single messages to give listeners a rough idea of the topic. Yes-no questions were still used to solve most communication breakdowns at the time of this writing.

Future Intervention

There are several aspects of Rhonda's intervention that are still before us. First, we hope to continue to broaden her use of the system. We would like to expand her vocabulary and add more overlays. Eventually, we hope to reduce the size of the symbols, place two levels on one overlay, and teach Rhonda to change the levels independently. We hope to train Rhonda in the use of interaction phrases and in initiation with the board. We would also like to provide her with some limited syntactic training in multiple word responses in sequences, as well as simple constructions for questions. We have taught Rhonda only at Vicker's (1974) presyntactic (one-word) programming level primarily because it is a level of use that is powerful for Rhonda. At this time, we feel it is essential to show her and her parents the power of the system in natural, albeit limited, communication. In addition, the Talking Word Board, if arranged well, can provide the syntactic structure where necessary, so the user does not have to be sophisticated in syntactic usage.

The second respect in which we plan to continue our intervention is in the development of a portable system. As discussed earlier, the Talking Word Board system utilizes an Apple II computer, which at this time is not portable. This means that Rhonda's training and communication take place in a single setting—e.g., at the dining room table. We are currently working with several commercial software companies to make the Talking Word Board compatible with a computer that could be mounted to a wheelchair. When such a system is available to Rhonda, we will continue with some intervention goals related to generalization of her communication skills and performance trials to evaluate the effectiveness of the system.

QUESTIONS FOR THE CLINICIAN

Question 1. How would your intervention be different if Rhonda were 4 years old at the time of your first evaluation?

Our approach to training would be quite different in several respects. First, all interaction would be in the context of age-appropriate play. Meyers (1983) used a system similar to the Talking Word Board with children as young as 2 years of age. She utilized play routines, such as singing and playing with objects that are familiar and reinforcing to the individual child. Meyers structures her training around those activities according to a number of principles, which she describes well in her 1983 article.

Second, we would provide Rhonda with a greater number of play opportunities above and beyond the communication system use. Carlson (personal communication) has described a number of ways to provide a physically disabled child with play activities. She has constructed boards, for example, that have slots to hold modified toys. The slots function as runners that permit the child to slide the toy but prevent it from falling to the floor, out of the child's reach. Musselwhite and Carlson (1983) have described a means of suspending toys in front of a child in a frame that permits changing the toys easily. Again, this allows the child to reach the toys easily while preventing them from falling out of reach. All such techniques would be utilized to increase the amount and diversity of play Rhonda could experience.

Third, our intervention would be more heavily directed towards Vicker's (1974) syntactic programming. We would eventually structure the Talking Word Board overlays more along the lines of Musselwhite and St. Louis's (1982) multiple simultaneous displays to facilitate this syntactic training. This would be coupled with reading recognition and spelling training at school. The goal would be to provide Rhonda with a communication approach that would complement, not distract from, the development of her knowledge of normal English structure.

Question 2. How can an individual's instruction on the Talking Word Board be integrated into daily communication interactions until a fully portable system becomes available?

The symbols used with the Talking Word Board are usually mounted on a sheet of thin, transparent plastic. If several symbol sets are used with a single individual, or if several different individuals use a symbol set, the plastic overlays can be changed rapidly. These overlays can also be used as traditional communication boards. If this approach is attempted, a means of protecting and transporting multiple overlays is necessary.

Several years ago we developed a multiple overlay communication board for one of our clients. Gary did not speak because of severe athetoid cerebral palsy; he was unable to read or spell. When he entered a cerebral palsy residential center, he was introduced to Blissymbols by his speech pathologist, Kathy Smith. After a couple of years, he had learned such a large number of these symbols that they could no longer be displayed on his laptray in such a way that he could see and accurately point to them. The decision was made to divide Gary's symbols and display them on several different communication board overlays. For example, one overlay was to contain general conversational messages. Another was to contain messages to be used in the sheltered workshop. As he continued to learn additional symbols, the number of overlays would increase.

In order to accommodate the multiple overlays, a special wheelchair laptray was constructed by Marvin Soderquist in our Engineering Applications Center. This board doubled as a communication board holder, which could hold as many as ten plastic communication overlays. The laptray, shown in Figure 13–3, was constructed of two sheets of three eighths inch Plexiglas with a compartment 0.5 inch wide sandwiched in between.

Gary communicated by pointing to the Blissymbols displayed on the top sheet (Fig. 13–4). The symbols were positioned on each of the plastic sheets in exactly the same locations, so that the symbols on the top sheet covered the symbols on the remaining sheets. The white circles were placed on the overlay to remind Gary to position his finger so that he did not obscure the symbol or the printed label. When he moved from setting to setting, the staff or his family members rearranged the plastic sheets, so that the appropriate symbols were displayed. Gary's overlay sheets were also coded with a colored tab in the upper left hand corner. Each overlay had these tabs representing each of the other overlay sheets. By pointing to a given tab, Gary could request that a specific overlay be moved to the top position.

Gary has used this communication board with three different overlays for several years. The multiple overlay approach has accommodated the variety of displays that is necessary for Gary. We had hoped that Gary would begin to use the Talking Word Board system. Recently, however, spinal arthritis has reduced Gary's range of arm movement, interfering significantly with this plan.

Question 3. You mention several symbol systems with regard to Rhonda. Which systems are most commonly used in the field of communication augmentation and how do they differ?

It is not possible for us to discuss all of the symbol systems that have been used in this field. The interested reader is referred to the

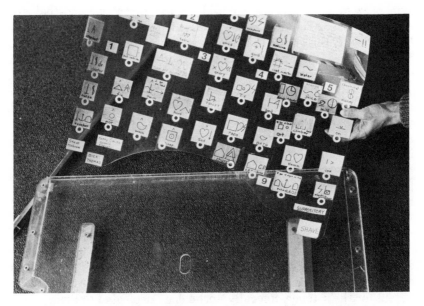

Figure 13-3. An overlay being inserted into Gary's laptray.

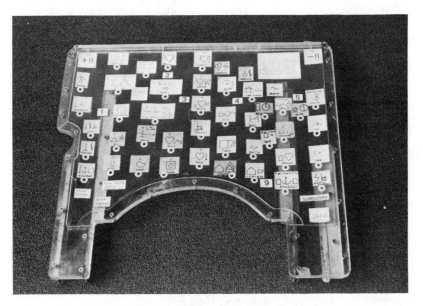

Figure 13-4. Gary's personal care overlay.

References and *Additional Readings* sections for a list of resources on symbol systems. However, we will discuss three systems that are commonly used. The first such system, Blissymbolics, was developed by Charles K. Bliss (1965) as an international communication system. The system was later adapted for use in communication augmentation at the Ontario Crippled Children's Centre (Kates and McNaughton, 1975). The Bliss approach utilizes a small number of basic shapes, alone or in combination, to represent meaning. Some of the symbols and combinations of symbols have a high symbolic load in that they bear an arbitrary relationship to the referent. Other symbols are more intelligible to untrained viewers because they are line drawings of their referents. In addition to shape, meaning is determined by the size, position, spacing and orientation of the symbols. The reader is referred back to Figure 13-2 for examples of such arbitrary and iconic symbols.

Initially, Blissymbols were used extensively on communication boards. As time passed, communication systems became more flexible; both the symbols used on the display and the messages programmed as output could be fully customized. This permitted the use of Blissymbols on the control display, paired with either printed or synthesized speech output for the listener. Recently, technology dedicated to Blissymbols has been developed. Kelso and Vanderheiden (1982) developed the BlissApple software program for use with Apple computers. This software contains a large dictionary of Blissymbols that can be included in the subroutines of communication augmentation systems to meet the individual cognitive and motor capabilities of the nonspeaking individual. Sheri Hunnicutt (personal communication), of the Royal Institute of Technology in Stockholm, has described a direct selection communication system with a Blissymbol control display. The output of the system is speech synthesis in French, English, or Swedish.

Another symbol system used with nonreading individuals was developed by Faith Carlson (1983). Picsyms are not so much a symbol set as a system for creating and using symbols for an individual nonspeaker. The development of the symbols is guided by many of the issues discussed earlier for Rhonda, including the symbolic load and semantic applicability of the symbols. Carlson also utilizes the salient characteristics (from the user's perspective) as symbols of particular objects, events, or people. For example, Figure 13-5 shows the symbol chosen to represent "Bobby Jo," a friend who wore sunglasses that were fascinating to the nonspeaking individual. The Picsyms approach is flexible in that it allows the rapid preparation of new symbols to communicate about ongoing events in the user's life. Initial work to combine the Picsym approach with computer technology has been reported by Carlson, Cohen, and Geiger (1982).

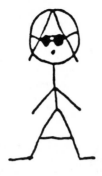

Bobby Jo

Figure 13-5. A Picsym representing some characteristics of a friend.

Recently, Prentke Romich has introduced a system which utilizes the Minspeak symbol approach. Minspeak, as developed by Bruce Baker (1982), is used as a means of encoding messages for ease of recall. In the Prentke Romich Minspeak system, the user selects a sequence of arbitrary symbols to represent each message stored for retrieval at another time. Individual users can employ different schemes to assign the symbols. For a specific example of the use of Minspeak, the reader is referred to Chapter 2.

REFERENCES

Baker, B. Minspeak. *Byte*, 1982, *7*; 186-203.

Bliss, C.K. *Semantography-Blissymbolics*. Sydney, Australia: Semantography Publications, 1965.

Carlson, F. Alternate methods of communication. In R. Forcucci (Ed.), *A handbook for students and clinicians*. Danville, IL: Interstate Printers and Publishers, 1981.

Carlson, F. *Picsyms workshop manual*. Omaha, NE: Meyer Children's Rehabilitation Institute, 1983.

Carlson, F.L., Cohen, C.G., and Geiger, C. The use of Picsyms with an Apple II microcomputer. Presentation at ASHA, Toronto, 1982.

Clark, C.R. Learning words using traditional orthography and the symbols of Rebus, Bliss, and Carrier. *Journal of Speech and Hearing Disorders*, 1981, *46*, 191-196.

Hughes, M.J. Sequencing of visual and auditory stimuli in teaching words and Bliss Symbols to the mentally retarded. *Australian Journal of Mental Retardation*, 1979, (5), 298-302.

Kates, B., and McNaughton, S. *The first application of Blissymbolics as a communication medium for non-speaking children: History and Development, 1971-1974*. Toronto, Ontario: Blissymbolics Communication Institute, 1975.

Kelso, D., and Vanderheiden, G. *BlissApple program*. Madison, WI: Trace Center, 1982.

Lloyd, L.L., and Karlan, G.R. Non-speech communication symbols and systems: Where have we been and where are we going? *Journal of Mental Deficiency Research*, 1984, *28*, 3-20.

McNaughton, S. and Kates, B. The application of Blissymbolics. In R.L. Schiefelbusch (Ed.), *Nonspeech Language and Communication: Analysis and Intervention*. Baltimore: University Park Press, 1980.

Meyers, L.F. Unique contributions of microcomputers to language intervention with handicapped children. *Seminars in Speech and Language*, 1983, *5*, 23-35.

Musselwhite, C.R. A comparison of three symbolic communication systems. Unpublished doctoral dissertation, West Virginia University, 1982.

Musselwhite, C.R. Visual communication systems for the nonreading nonspeaker. In the proceedings of an augmentative communication conference entitled *Working with prereaders: practical approaches*), March 3-4, 1983. Proceedings are available from Meyer Children's Rehabilitation Institute, University of Nebraska Medical Center, Omaha, Nebraska, 68131.

Musselwhite, C.R., and Carlson, F. Adaptive play as a preliminary communication strategy for nonspeaking children. ASHA, 1983, *25*, 61.

Musselwhite, C.R., and St. Louis, K.W. *Communication programming for the severely handicapped: Vocal and non-vocal strategies*. San Diego: College-Hill Press, 1982.

Vicker, B. Communication board programming with a four-year-old child: A case report. In B. Vicker (Ed.), *Nonoral communication system project 1964-1973*. Iowa City, IA: Campus Stores, Publishers, 1974.

ADDITIONAL READINGS

Albert, C. Procedures for determining the optimal nonspeech mode with the autistic child. In R.L. Schiefelbusch (Ed.), *Nonspeech Language and Communication: Analysis and intervention*. Baltimore: University Park Press, 1980.

Archer, L.A. Blissymbolics – a nonverbal communication system. *Journal of Speech and Hearing Disorders*, 1977,*42*; 568-579.

Blau, A.F. Vocabulary selection in augmentative communication: Where do we begin. In H. Winitz (Ed.), *For clinicians by clinicians: Language disorders*. Baltimore: University Park Press, 1983.

Bonvillian, J.D., Nelson, K.E., and Rhyne, J.M. Sign language and autism. *Journal of Autism and Developmental Disabilities*, 1982, *11*, 125-138.

Calculator, S., and Dollaghan, C. The use of communication boards in a residential setting: An evaluation. *Journal of Speech and Hearing Disorders*, 1982, *47*, 281-287.

Carlson, F. A format for selecting vocabulary for the nonspeaking child. *Language, Speech and Hearing Services in the Schools*, 1981, *12*, 240-245.

Carrier, J.K. Nonspeech noun usage training with severely and profoundly retarded children. *Journal of Speech and Hearing Research*, 1974, *14*, 510-517.

Carrier, J.K., Jr. Application of a nonspeech language system with the severely language handicapped. In L.L. Lloyd (Ed.), *Communication Assessment and Intervention Strategies*. Baltimore: University Park Press, 1976.

Cohen, M.S., Jones, K.L., and Deal L.K. Blissymbolics: Can't talk doesn't have to mean can't communicate. ASHA 1979, *21*, 779.

Finke, J.A. Homage to Blissymbolics: Pictographic language opens the world to persons with communication disabilities. *Rehabilitation World*. 1980, *5*(4), 30-33.

Fristoe, M., and Lloyd, L. A survey of the use of non-speech communication systems with the severely communication impaired. *Mental Retardation*. 1978, *16*, 99-103.

Fristoe, M. and Lloyd, L.L. Planning an initial expressive sign lexicon for persons with severe communication impairment. *Journal of Speech and Hearing Disorders*, 1980, *45*, 170-180.

Griffith, P.L. and Robinson, J.H. Influence of iconicity and phonological similarity on sign learning by mentally retarded children. *American Journal of Mental Deficiency* 1980, *85*(3), 291-298.

Harris, D. Communication interaction processes involving nonvocal physically handicapped children. *Topics in Language Disorders*, 1982, *2*, 21-37.

Harris, D., Brown, W.P., McKenzie, P., Riener, S., and Scheibel, C. Symbol communication for the mentally handicapped. *Mental Retardation*. 1975, *13*(1).

Harris, D., Lippert, J., Yoder, D., Vanderheiden, G. Blissymbols: An augmentative symbol communication system for nonvocal severely handicapped children. In R. York and E. Edgar (Eds.), *Teaching the Severely Handicapped* (Vol 4). Columbus, OH: Special Press, 1979.

Harris, D., Vanderheiden, G. Enhancing communicative interaction skills in nonvocal severely physically handicapped children. In R.L. Schiefelbusch (Ed.), *Nonspeech Language Intervention*. Baltimore: University Park Press, 1980.

Harris-Vanderheiden, D. Blissymbols and the mentally retarded. In G.C. Vanderheiden and K. Grilley (Eds.), *Non-Vocal Communication Techniques and Aids for the Severely Physically Handicapped*. Baltimore: University Park Press, 1976.

Kreigsman, E., Gallaher, J. and Meyers, A. Sign programs with non-verbal hearing children. *Exceptional Children*, 1982, *48*, 436-445.

Lancioni, G. E. Using pictorial representations as communication means with low-functioning children. *Journal of Autism and Developmental Disorders*, 1983, *13*, 87-105.

McLean, L., and McLean, J.E. A language training program for nonverbal autistic children. *Journal of Speech and Hearing Disorders*, 1974, *39*, 186-193.

Morris, S.E. Communication interaction development at mealtimes for the multiply handicapped child: Implications for the use of augmentative communication systems. *Language Speech and Hearing Services in the Schools*, 1981, *12*, 216-232.

Rosegrant, T.J. Fostering progress in literacy development: Technology and social interaction. *Seminars in Speech and Language*, 1984, *5*, 47-58.

Schiefelbusch, R.L, (Ed.). *Nonspeech Language and Communication: Analysis and intervention*. Baltimore: University Park Press, 1980.

Schuler, A.L., Baldwin, M. Nonspeech communication and childhood autism. *Language Speech and Hearing Services in the Schools*. 1981, *12*, 246-257.

Shane, H.C., Lipschultz, R.W., and Shane, C.L. Facilitating the communicative interaction of nonspeaking persons in large residential settings. *Topics in Language Disorders*. 1982, *2*, 73-84.

Shane, H.C., and Wilbur, R.B. Potential for expressive signing based on motor control. *Sign Language Studies*, 1980, *29*, 331-347.

Shane, H.C. and Wilson, M.S. Blissymbols. *ASHA*, 1977, *19*, 223.

Wilbur, R. B. Nonspeech symbol systems. In R.L. Schiefelbusch (Ed.), *Nonspeech Language and Communication: Analysis and Intervention*. Baltimore: University Park Press, 1980.

Yoder, D.E., Calculator, S. Some perspectives on intervention strategies for persons with developmental disorders. *Journal of Autism and Developmental Disabilities*, 1981, *11*(1), 107–123.

Yorkston, K.M., and Dowden, P.A. Nonspeech language and communication systems. In A. Holland (Ed.), *Language disorders in adults: Recent advances*: San Diego: College-Hill Press, 1984, pp. 284-312.

GLOSSARY

Adaptive Firmware Card A card for the Apple II+ or IIe computer that allows physically disabled individuals who are unable to operate a standard keyboard to run off-the-self software using 10 different input methods. The card allows the computer to be controlled through Morse code, such that most conventional Apple compatible software can be controlled through one or two switch Morse code rather than from the keyboard only (see Chapters 3 and 6). The card also allows the Apple computer to be controlled through a linear scan function, which is displayed along the bottom on the computer monitor. With this function, the Apple computer can be controlled with one switch scanning rather than keyboard only. An additional card function allows the "one-finger typist" to "lock" the shift and control functions so they can be managed with one finger. The card also allows the Apple computer to receive ASCII code from other computers or peripherals, such as the Unicorn keyboard. In addition the card also allows the game playing function described in Chapter 10. (For a more detailed discussion, see Schwejda, P., and Vanderheiden, G. Adaptive firmware card for the Apple II. *Byte*, 1982, 7, 276–317. The adaptive Firmware Card is manufactured and distributed by Adaptive Peripherals, 4529 Bagley Ave. N., Seattle, WA 98103.)

Adduct To pull or draw toward midline.

ADL Activities of daily living.

Amyotrophic lateral sclerosis (ALS) A degenerative disease resulting in degeneration of the nuclei of upper and lower motor neurons.

Anarthria Severe dysarthria resulting in speechlessness.

Anoxia Deprivation of oxygen to the brain.

Aphasia A language impairment due to central nervous system damage.

Apraxia of speech An articulatory disorder resulting from impairment of the capacity to position of the muscles of speech and follow the sequence of muscle movements needed for the volitional production of phonemes. The speech musculature does not show significant weakness, slowness, or incoordination when used for reflexive, automatic acts.

ASCII An acronym for the American Standard Code for Information Interchange. This standard code assigns a unique value from 0 to 127 to each of 128 numbers, letters, special characters, and control characters.

Aspiration The penetration of food or liquid into the respiratory system.

Assessment of Intelligibility of Dysarthric Speech A standardized test of single word and sentence intelligibility, speaking rate, and communication efficiency. (Published by C.C. Publications, Inc., Tigard, OR 97005, 1981.)

Asymmetric tonic neck reflex (ATNR) A reflex consisting of extension of the arm and sometimes the leg on the side to which the head is turned, with flexion of the contralateral limbs.

Athetoid cerebral palsy A motor impairment with frequent, involuntary, writhing movements.

A-Tronix Morse code translator A device that translates Morse code into English. (Manufactured by A-Tronix, Suite 6, 23151 Alcade Drive, Laguna Hills, CA 92653.) (See Chapters 3 and 6.)

Blissymbols A symbol set initially developed for intercultural communication but later adopted for communication in nonreading disabled populations. The Bliss approach utilizes a consistent set of symbols to represent common meaning. (For further information, see Chapter 13 and McNaughton, S., and Kates, B. The application of blissymbolics. In R. L. Schiefelbusch [*Ed.*], *Nonspeech language and communication: Analysis and intervention.* Baltimore, University Park Press, 1980.)

BSR An environmental control system with control module and peripheral modules that can be inserted into conventional electrical outlets. The system allows remote control of electrical devices.

Canon Communicator A portable tape typewriter. (Distributed in the United States by Telesensory, Inc., Palo Alto, CA, and Prentke Romich, Company, Shreve, OH 44676-9421.)

Capability assessment A process completed during the evaluation in which the motor control, language, cognitive, visual, and hearing capabilities of the individual are assessed.

Categories Test A subtest of the Halsted Reitan Battery, which measures abstracting ability in which figures of varying size, shape, number, intensity, color, and location are grouped by abstract principles. Subjects identify the principle by responding on a simple keyboard. (See Halsted, W. C. *Brain and language*. Chicago: University of Chicago Press, 1947; Reitan, R. M., and Davidson, L. A. *Clinical neuropsychology: Current status and application*. New York: Winston/Wiley, 1974.)

Cerebral palsy Motor paralysis, paresis, or incoordination occurring as a result of damage to the brain at or near the time of birth; often associated with perceptual, sensory, and cognitive disorders.

Cerebrovascular accident (CVA or stroke) Brain tissue damage owing to deprivation of bloodflow secondary to hemorrhage or occlusion of an artery.

Computer-based communication augmentation system A device or approach hosted by a computer and used to augment or provide an alternative to human speech.

Control display The display on a communication augmentation system employed by the user to observe message choices and monitor the status of message preparation.

Conversational control The manner and extent to which an individual directs or restrains communication interaction. It represents a broad range of behaviors that occur in interaction, including obtaining and maintaining turns, initiating topics, interrupting a partner's turn, and changing roles from responder to initiator.

Cortical blindness Severe visual impairment owing to a lesion of the primary visual cortex.

Dedicated system A device utilized for only one application, such as communication.

Direct selection A control strategy for a communication augmentation system in which the user can activate any of the choices presented on the control display.

Directed Scanning See *Scanning*.

Dysarthria A group of motor speech disorders resulting from disturbances in muscular control — weakness, slowness, or incoordination — of the speech mechanism owing to damage to the central or peripheral nervous system.

Electrolarynx A device used by laryngectomized individuals to produce sound for speech. (See Chapters 6 and 9.)

Environmental control unit (ECU) A device that permits control of numerous electrically powered appliances, e.g., lights, fan, door-opener, and so forth, with single or multiple switches.

Epson HX-20 computer A small, portable, battery-powered computer with built-in miniprinter, screen, and microcassette that is distributed through local computer stores. (See Chapters 5 and 8.)

Express communication system(s) A "family" of communication systems with multiple interface options, including several direct selection and scanning approaches. Messages can be selected through letter-by-letter spelling or message retrieval. Messages can be programmed in the field by the user or another adult. Output options include print and speech synthesis options. (Manufactured by Prentke Romich Company, Shreve, OH 44676-9421.)

Extension The act of straightening or extending a limb.

Eye-gaze A strategy of communication augmentation in which choices are indicated by gazing at the preferred object or symbol.

Flaccidity Weak, lax, and soft.

Flexion The act of bending or being bent.

Gates-MacGinitie Reading Test Standardized reading test with levels ranging from early elementary through college. Responses are indicated in multiple-choice format.

(Published by Teacher's College Press, Columbia University, New York, NY.)
Glossectomy Surgical removal of part or all of the tongue.
Handivoice 130 A communication augmentation device that requires direct selection interface and features speech synthesis output. Messages in the form of single words, phrases, single letters or numbers, and sounds can be retrieved and combined. (Manufactured and distributed by Phonic Ear, Inc., 250 Camino Alto, Mill Valley, CA 94941.) (See Chapter 12.)
Hardware The physical parts of a computer.
Headlight pointer A device that emits a focused light beam used by a physically handicapped individual to indicate communication choices.
Illinois Test of Psycholinguistic Abilities (ITPA) A standardized test of linguistic and related abilities. (Published by University of Illinois Institute for Research on Exceptional Children, Urbana, IL 61801, 1961.)
Interface A general term refering to the manner and strategy employed by physically disabled individuals to control a communication augmentation device.
Interrupted scanning See *Scanning.*
Keyboard emulator An alternative means of accessing a computer when keyboard control is not possible.
Laptray A tray attached to a wheelchair.
Laryngectomy Surgical removal of all or part of the larynx.
Latching switch A switch that locks into a "closed" or "open" position, such as a light switch.
LED Light emitting diode.
Lexicon A vocabulary or stock of words used in a particular profession, subject, or style.
Lower extremities Legs and feet.
Mainstreaming The inclusion of disabled students in the educational experience and environment of nondisabled students.
Melodic Intonation Therapy A therapy approach in which speech production is encouraged by pairing speech with melodic patterns. (See Chapter 12.)
Membrane keys An interface with a flat, continuous surface; individual switches are activated by pressure.
Message retrieval The process by which entire messages can be elicited in response to a short code.
Minspeak A strategy for addressing and retrieving messages by means of a sequence of symbols. (Available through Prentke Romich, Shreve, OH 44676-9421.) (See Chapter 2.)
Modem A device that permits intercomputer or monitor-computer communication over a telephone line.
Momentary switch A switch that is "open" or "closed" only when the switch is activated.
Morse code A system of communication in which alphabet letters and numbers are represented by short and long patterns of sound or light. (See Chapters 3, 6, and 10.)
Motor learning Developing an understanding of the consequences of motor activity, including interface control. (See Chapter 4.)
Needs assessment An evaluation of the communication needs of a nonspeaking individual or one with a severe communication disorder, in which a specific list is compiled of the communication tasks that are mandatory or desirable for the individual.
Neck dissection A surgical procedure by which lymphatic tissue is removed from the neck.
Overlay A sheet, usually of plastic, on which pictures, symbols, and messages are mounted to be used as a control display for a communication augmentation approach.
Optical headpointer The head-mounted optical interface utilized with the Express communication system(s). (See Chapter 2.)
PACE (Promoting Aphasics, Communicative Effectiveness) Therapy A therapy approach for aphasic individuals in which the development of communication interaction skills is stressed.
Peabody Picture Vocabulary Test A test of receptive vocabulary with a multiple-choice response format. (Published by American Guidance Services, Circle Pines, MN 55014, 1965.)

Peabody Individual Achievement Test   A test of a number of academic skills, including spelling recognition, reading, and mathematics, administered in a multiple-choice format. (Published by American Guidance Services, Circle Pines, MN 55014, 1970.)

Pectoral flaps   Tissue with its blood supply from the pectoral area, which is positioned to fill the defect resulting from surgery for oropharyngeal cancer.

Phrenic nerve pacer   A device which stimulates the phrenic nerves to accomplish respiratory function in selected individuals with paralysis of the diaphragm owing to a spinal cord lesion above the nuclei of the phrenic nerves. (See Chapter 6.)

Picsyms   Line-drawing symbols that represent concepts, actvities, persons, characteristics, or places. (See Chapter 13 for a discussion of various symbol sets.)

Program   A sequence of instructions that describes a process for a computer.

Porch Index of Communicative Abilities (PICA)   A test of communication performance used primarily with aphasic individuals. (Published by Consulting Psychologists Press, Palo Alto, CA 94306, 1967.)

Raven's Progressive Matrices Test   A nonverbal intelligence test with a multiple-choice response format. (Published by H. K. Lewis, London, England.)

RAM (random access memory)   The main memory of a computer. The computer can store values in distinct locations in RAM and recall them again, or alter and restore them.

Reading recognition   The ability to recognize words from a graphic presentation only.

Rebus   A symbol set used for communication by nonreading individuals. (See Chapter 13 for a discussion of various symbol sets.)

ROM (read only memory)   This type of memory is usually used to hold important programs or data that must be available to the computer when the power is first turned on. Information in ROM is placed there in the process of manufacturing the ROM and is unalterable.

Row-column scanning   See *Scanning.*

Respirator-dependent   Unable to support oneself respiratorily without the aid of a respirator (ventilator).

Quadriplegia   Paralysis of all four limbs.

Scanning   Selections are offered to the user in a variety of modes. In the *linear mode,* all of the selections are offered sequentially and the user interrupts the process to select a location that contains the desired letter, symbol, picture, or words. In the *row-column mode,* selections are offered by scanning down the rows until the user interrupts the scan, and then selections are offered by scanning across the rows until the user interrupts the scan at the desired location. In the *directed scanning mode,* the scanning process is under the control of the user's interface. The user activates multiple switches or a joystick to direct the scanning cursor to the desired location.

ScanWRITER   A communication augmentation device in which row-column scanning and directed scanning are used as interface strategies. Single letters or entire words or phrases can be retrieved. Output is printed or spoken with a speech synthesizer. The device is also a keyboard emulator or the Apple II + and IIe computers. (Manufactured and distributed by Zygo Industries, Inc., P.O. Box 1008, Portland, OR 97197-1008.) (See Chapter 11.)

Scoliosis   A lateral deviation of the normally straight vertical axis of the spine.

Sharp Memowriter   A "family" of communication augmentation devices that allow letter-by-letter spelling, limited message retrieval, and calculation. Output appears on a marquee display and a printer. (Distributed by Sharp, Paramus, NJ 07652.) (See Chapter 8.)

Sharp Expanded Keyboard Memowriter   A Sharp Memowriter only with an expanded keyboard. (Distributed by Prentke Romich Company, Shreve, OH 44676-4421.)

Sip-and-puff switch   A two switch interface; one switch is activated with negative air pressure and the other is activated with positive air pressure.

Software   The programs that may be loaded into the computer and direct its functions.

Spastic cerebral palsy   A persistent motor impairment appearing before the age of 3 years, owing to nonprogressive brain damage with hypertonic muscles, resulting in stiffness and slowness of movement.

Spinal cord lesion   Damage to the spinal cord.
Symbolic load   The extent to which a gesture is an arbitrary symbol for the concept it conveys.
Synthesized speech   Speech produced with a computer.
Test of Auditory Comprehension of Language   A standardized test of various language structures with multiple-choice response format. (Published by Learning Concepts, Austin, TX.)
Text-to-speech algorithm   A computer algorithm that translates standard orthographic into spoken messages.
Tracheostomy   A surgical incision of the trachea through the skin and muscles of the anterior neck.
Tracheostomy tube   A plastic or metal tube inserted through the tracheotomy into the trachea. The tube serves to keep the tracheotomy from closing naturally and as a guide for insert of a suctioning tube into the trachea.
Upper extremities   Arms and hands.
Vocaid   A communication augmentation device with synthesized speech ouput and direct selection interface. (Manufactured by Texas Instruments, Lubbock, TX 79408.)
Wechsler Adult Intelligence Scale (WAIS)   An individually administered composite test battery including 11 subtests. Results are reported as Full Scale, Verbal, and Performance IQ scores. (Published by Psychological Corporation, New York, NY.)
Wheelchair laptray   See *Laptray*.
Wide Range Achievement Test   A standardized test measuring a variety of academic performance areas. (Published by Guidance Associates, Wilmington, DE.)
Zygo 16 row-column scanner   A communication augmentation device activated with a single switch in direct and interrupted scanning modes. (Manufactured by Zygo Industries, Inc., P.O. Box 1008, Portland, OR 97297-1008.)

APPENDIX I

NEEDS ASSESSMENT

AUGMENTATIVE COMMUNICATION CENTER
DEPARTMENT OF REHABILITATION MEDICINE
UNIVERSITY OF WASHINGTON HOSPITAL

Name:

Date:

Interviewer:

Responders:

Please indicate whether the needs listed are:
    M – Mandatory
    D – Desirable
    U – Unimportant
    F – May be mandatory in the future

Positioning

In bed:
    While supine
    While lying prone
    While lying on side
    While in a Clinitron bed
    While in a Roto bed
    While sitting in bed
    While in arm restraints
    In a variety of positions

Related to mobility:
    Carry the system while walking
    Independently position the system
    In a manually controlled wheelchair
    In an electric wheelchair
    With a lapboard
    While the chair is reclined
    Arm troughs

Other equipment:
    With hand mitts
    With arterial lines
    Orally intubated
    While trached
    With oxygen mask
    With electric wheelchair controls
    Environmental control units

Other needs related to positioning:

Communication Partners

Someone who cannot read (e.g., child or nonreader)
Someone with no familiarity with the system
Someone who has poor vision
Someone who has limited time or patience
Someone who is across the room or in another room
Someone who is not independently mobile
Several people at a time
Someone who is hearing impaired

Other needs related to partners:

Locations

Only in a single room
In multiple rooms with the same building
In dimly lit rooms
In bright rooms
In noisy rooms
Outdoors
While traveling in a car, van, and so forth
While moving from place to place within a building
At a desk or computer terminal
In more than two locations in a day

Other needs related to locations:

Message Needs

Call attention
Signal emergencies
Answer yes-no questions
Provide unique information
Make requests
Carry on a conversation
Express emotion
Give opinions
Convey basic medical needs
Greet people
Prepare messages in advance
Edit texts written by others
Edit texts prepared by the user
Make changes in diagrams
Compile lists (e.g., phone numbers)
Perform calculations
Take notes

Other needs related to messages:

Modality Of Communication

Prepare printed messages
Prepare auditory messages
Talk on the phone
Communicate with other equipment (e.g., environment control
units)
Communicate privately with some partners
Switch from one modality to another during communication
Via several modalities at a time
(e.g., taking notes while talking on the phone)
Communicate via an intercom
Via formal letters or reports
On pre-prepare worksheets

Other needs related to modality of communication:

APPENDIX II

AUGMENTATIVE COMMUNICATION EVALUATION
INTAKE INFORMATION

I. IDENTIFYING INFORMATION

Name: _____ Birthdate: _____

Street Address: _____ Today's Date: _____

City, State, Zip: _____ Age: _____

Phone: _____ Referred By: _____

Parent or Guardian name　　　　　Address　　　　　Phone
(if applicable)

Physician name　　　　　Address　　　　　Phone

School/Workshop/Hospital name　　　　　Address　　　　　Phone

Contact Person School/Workshop or Hospital　　　　　Phone

Describe current communication problem as fully as possible: _____

II. PHYSICAL/MEDICAL FACTORS

Medical condition/diagnosis? _____ Onset? _____

Seizures? _____ Medications? _____

Ambulates? _____ Assisted? _____ With what? _____

Uses a wheelchair? _____ Power or Manual? _____

Type of Chair? _____ Wheelchair Control? _____

Feeds self? _____ Assisted? _____ With what? _____

Visual acuity? _____ Perception? _____ Aid? _____

Date of most recent exam? _____

Hearing acuity? _____ Perception? _____ Aid? _____

Date of most recent exam? _____

*From Non Oral Communication Assessment Forms, Non Oral Communication Center,
Plavan School, Fountain Valley, CA, 1980.

II. Physical/Medical Factors (Cont'd)

Gross Motor Control? _____

_____

Fine Motor Control?_____

_____

What is his/her most reliable motor actions? (i.e. raising arm, pointing, eye gaze, turning head, etc.)

1. _____

2. _____

3. _____

III. ACADEMIC/COGNITIVE FACTORS

Years of school completed _____High school grade equivalent? _____

Mental Age_____ Test_____Date_____Valid?_____

Subjects or area of interest? _____

Grade in school/class placement (i.e. severely handicapped, physically handicapped, etc.) _____

_____

_____

Specific future educational plans:
  Next year: _____

  In five years: _____

Comments: _____

_____

IV. VOCATIONAL/AVOCATIONAL FACTORS

List his/her most recent vocational activities, duties, and dates:

	Position	Duties	Dates
1.	_____	_____	_____ to _____
2.	_____	_____	_____ to _____
3.	_____	_____	_____ to _____

IV. Vocational/Avocational Factors (Cont'd)

List his/her future vocational plans:

    Position   Duties

_____   _____

_____   _____

List his/her avocational interests:

_____

_____

If test scores are unavailable, please provide the following:

Functional reading vocabulary: _____

_____

_____

Functional spelling vocabulary: _____

_____

_____

V. COMMUNICATION FACTORS

How does he/she communicate now?

At home? _____

_____

At school? _____

_____

At work? _____

_____

Does he/she understand the speech of others?	YES	NO
Does he/she follow directions?	YES	NO
Does he/she make wants known?	YES	NO
Does he/she initiate communication?	YES	NO

V. Communication Factors (Cont'd)

Does he/she speak in words at times?   YES   NO

Does he/she make sounds?   YES   NO

Does he/she indicate yes and no appropriately?   YES   NO

Does he/she use facial expression?   YES   NO

Does he/she use body language?   YES   NO

How do you know when he/she wishes to communicate? _____

Communication system previously (i.e., board, electronic/mechanical aid, signing, etc.) _____

Receptive Language Score _____Instrument Used _____Date _____

_____   _____   _____

Expressive Language
Score   _____Instrument Used _____Date _____

_____   _____   _____

Read Score   _____Instrument Used _____Date _____

_____   _____   _____

Spelling Score   _____Instrument Used _____Date _____

_____   _____   _____

VI. ENVIRONMENTAL NEEDS

What percentage of a typical day is spent in:

Wheelchair	_____ %	Home	_____ %
Walker	_____ %	Job	_____ %
Lying down	_____ %	School	_____ %
Other	_____ %	Bus/Traveling	_____ %
Indoors	_____ %	Outdoors	_____ %

What changes in wheelchair seating are planned in the next year?_____

_____

VII. OTHER PROGRAMS

List professions from whom he/she is currently receiving therapy or instruction:

Name   Type of Therapy or Instruction

_____   _____

_____   _____

_____   _____

VII. FUNDING

Please indicate funding source for the evaluation: _____

If Medicaid, please enclose a valid medical coupon: _____

Author Index

Subject Index